DICK

For Alan and Chris—thanks for all the fun

DICK

A User's Guide

Michele Moore, M.D., FAAFP &
Caroline de Costa, M.B., B.S., FRANZCOG

Marlowe & Company
New York

DICK: *A User's Guide*

Copyright © 2003 Dr. Michele Moore and Dr. Caroline de Costa

Published by
Marlowe & Company
An Imprint of Avalon Publishing Group Incorporated
245 West 17th Street, 11th Floor
New York, NY 10011

Originally published in Australia by Allen & Unwin.
This edition published by arrangement.

Library of Congress Control Number: 2003113875

ISBN 1-56924-429-4

9 8 7 6 5 4 3 2 1

Designed by Pauline Neuwirth, Neuwirth and Associates, Inc.
Printed in the United States of America
Distributed by Publishers Group West

CONTENTS

FIGURES

ACKNOWLEDGMENTS

We would like to thank our agent Cleo Pozzo for her advice, editors Emma Cant and Alex Nahlous, and their staff for their invaluable contributions to our dicktionary, Tony Hillier, who read the manuscript and Javed de Costa for assistance with word processing. We are particularly grateful to our urologist colleague Dr. Arthur Cohen, who gave us the benefit of his many years of experience in pecker-checking.

Their support enabled us to keep it up, so to speak, when our spirits drooped, and ultimately to give it our best shot.

INTRODUCTION: STRAIGHT TALK

General and Madame de Gaulle were known for summering each year in the west of Ireland. They were also known for not giving interviews. However, as the story goes, a young woman reporter from the Irish Times *managed to set up an interview with Madame. The General was dozing by the fire in an adjacent room. After talking about the greatness of France and Madame's recipe for Crepes Suzette, the reporter asked: "Madame, what brings you to Ireland each year?" "Ah," replied Madame. "My dear, it is for a penis." The reporter could not believe her ears, and blushingly asked her to repeat this. "Yes," said Madame emphatically, "for a penis!" At this point the General woke up and called: "Non, non, cherie, how many times must I tell you! The word is ' 'appiness.' "*

Is this true? We hope so . . .

Why on earth would two *women* be writing a book about the penis? The answer is quite simple. We are both doctors working in the field of women's health, with more than fifty years' experience between us. Every day, we have conversations with women about their most intimate problems, their anatomy and its functioning, and their relationships with their partners. Often we talk with those partners too. And, despite the fact that sex is now quite freely discussed, and that since the 1960s women's sexuality has been liberated from the fear of unwanted pregnancy, we have been impressed by how often both women and men lack basic information about their bodies—about their own anatomy and how it functions. Misinformation abounds and there is certainly a dearth of good information about that most friendly male appendage, the penis.

The main thrust (ahem) of our argument is that, for most people, sex is inextricably linked with a penis—yet there is no accompanying guide book. The only source for needed information may be the media, and the information imparted—dare we say, inseminated?—may be inappropriate or even erroneous. Our correction of this lack of accurate information is not intended to be in any way disrespectful or salacious, but rather informative, fun, and titillating. Whether in marriage or in long- or short-term relationships, *everyone* has a need to know about the possible difficulties they or their partners may experience with the penis, so that they can be sensitive to their partners' needs, protect themselves from possible disease, and know when they or their partners need professional help.

Quite understandably, men are very fond of their penises, for which they have many slang names—including treasures ("the family jewels"), military metaphors (bayonets and swords), terms of formal address ("Captain!"), endearments ("big boy") and nicknames (Roger, Junior, and Johnson). And of course we can't forget Dick, which we like, and which you'll find popping up throughout our text. However, many men are curiously reluctant to openly discuss their penises in an informational way, although they may be very quick with jokes. (Heard about the shipment of Viagra that went missing at the city docks? The police are looking for a band of hardened criminals ... OK, we'll stop right there, but you see what we mean.) Little boys (and girls) quickly learn slang names—noodle, hose, wee wee, pee pee—for the penis, although they know the correct words for all the other parts of the body, and they soon get the idea that talking about "that" just isn't "nice." And after recently attending a showing of the paintings of Alice Neel, who has depicted several anatomically correct full-frontal nudes of men, as well as many other subjects, we found the men in our group were actually more impacted by the male nudes than were the women! (But then, wasn't it men who put all those fig leaves on statues?)

So this book has been written for *everyone* with an interest in the penis, from teenagers to nonagenarians ...

Prime-time TV and mainstream movies nearly always include a sexual theme. Sex sells—after all, people are interested in it. But it follows a formula. The lights dim, violins play, and he and she sink onto the nearest bed, couch, or sand dune. We might see a breast or buttock, catch a glimpse of pubic hair, but never anything remotely resembling a penis, let alone an upstanding one. Even *The Full Monty* was remarkable for the complete absence of its principal character. There is never any suggestion that a condom is being rolled on, or that erectile dysfunction or premature ejaculation might be a problem (that's not getting it up, and coming too quickly, respectively, and you'll be glad to learn that it's words like these—and not medical terms—that we try to use in this book). There are unwritten rules for most movies that are very carefully followed, and their effect is to deny their millions of viewers knowledge about what is normal, what actually happens in real life, and what can—and does—go wrong with the penis and the way it works. The same is true of the stereotyped videos that accompany almost all music now—easy sex, no information. Even when it comes to pornography, in magazines or on film (and let's face it, many adults do enjoy porn from time to time, on their own or together), though the penis is well displayed, it never droops, drips, or itches. And try putting the word "penis" into an Internet search: you will be rewarded with thousands of sites telling you how to make it bigger, but hardly a single one on basic anatomy, or condom use, or what to do if it's got spots on it. One important result of this lack of accurate information is that many people, young and old, still practice unsafe sex.

This book will give you information on the anatomy and functions of the penis, conditions that affect the appearance of the penis, and how these may affect a man's partners, circumcision, hygiene, condoms, sexually transmitted diseases, vasectomy, impotence, premature ejaculation, discharges, and some diseases of the penis and its appendages. It will also address some common myths, like the importance of penis size. At the end of the book, we provide as many of the slang or common usage terms as possible—nearly 400 in fact, and we have used many of these in our text. As a young woman, one of us was very embarrassed to find out that she had been using a "dirty" term as slang for something else. She misunderstood the connotation in which she heard the word used and thought it referred to someone not very bright. The real meaning was an artificial penis. Hopefully, the information in this book will spare you such awkwardness!

Our husbands have intimated that this is a "ballsy" undertaking for a couple of women, doctors or not, but so be it. "Ballsy" women, like men with balls, need accurate information . . . and, yes, we will also give you some information about the "balls": the scrotum and testes, and epididymis. We'll do this, whenever we can, with the help of some real-life stories from our own practices—the names and places have, of course, been changed. To give you some examples . . .

> Craig is a first-year lawyer in a large law firm. He recently met Meaghan, a receptionist at the firm, and they've been dating for about a month. In the past week, Craig and Meaghan have had sex several times. Meaghan is a contemporary woman and has always practiced safe sex; she sweetens the deal by very sensuously putting the condom on her partner as part of foreplay. The trouble is, the last time she did this for Craig, she thought she saw some funny bumps on his penis. Sophisticated though she may think she is, Meaghan has actually had only one other partner and she feels very shy about mentioning these bumps to Craig. She likes him a lot and she has to see him at work every day—what if he just walked out on her?

> Tony and Maria are in their early thirties. They've been married for eight years and have two children. In her last pregnancy, Maria had blood clots in her legs and lung and she was told not to get pregnant

again. She also was told that she couldn't take the Pill because of the clots. Both of her children were born by Caesarean section and Tony has said that now it's his turn to have surgery—after all, it's only a minor procedure for him. However, he just keeps putting it off—he's heard that "it makes you unable to get it up" and might cause a heart attack. Maria doesn't want any of that to happen, but she's also scared to death of getting pregnant again so she "has a headache" almost every night. He clams up when she tries to talk with him and now they're snarling at each other over whose turn it is to collect the kids from day care.

Evie is fifty-two and has been divorced since she was forty. Last Easter, she went on a tour to the wine country and met Fred. They've had a really nice time ever since, but it was a kind of old-fashioned romance until last week. After an early evening concert at one of their churches, Evie and Fred stopped at Nick's, a local bar, and had more than a few. They went back to Evie's house and one thing led to another. Everything was great right up to the crucial moment and then Fred just couldn't do it . . . He left in a hurry and hasn't called since or taken her calls. Evie's worried, feeling she did something wrong and maybe he found her repulsive and unattractive. As for Fred, he's just as miserable, but is too embarrassed to call her . . .

These and many other common scenarios will be outlined in this book and will be discussed without stigma or embarrassment. Being based on our own experience, and on discussions with the men and women we've cared for, the book is largely addressed to those in heterosexual relationships, whether casual or long-term. However, we hope that much of the general information we provide will also be of interest to gay men. So for everybody from age fifteen to ninety, whether you are the possessor of a penis or on the receiving end, whether you are young and free and out clubbing every night, or a new parent powdering a penis and wondering about circumcision, this is the book with the answers.

2 ANATOMY— OR HOW IT HANGS

The penis is a fleshy appendage that curls like a snail against the lower part of a man's abdomen. At least that is how it looks in its flaccid, limp state. When a man is sexually excited, this little snail lengthens and thickens and sticks out at an upward angle from the belly—it is then hard and rigid—a "bone."

There are in fact no bones in the penis of the human, or of any other animal—apart, it seems, from the possum (a little hard on the female possum, we think). Nor does the penis contain any voluntary muscles—claims that Dick is a muscle like the biceps needing regular exercise to prevent him wasting away have no basis in anatomy!

The penis was first methodically dissected and described by various Italian anatomists in the sixteenth century, including Fallopius and Vesalius, and accurate drawings of its inner and outer parts exist from that time.

The big banana consists basically of three cylinders or tubes of tissue. These are arranged with two cylinders on top (as you look down on the penis) and one on the bottom. These cylinders are roughly the size and shape

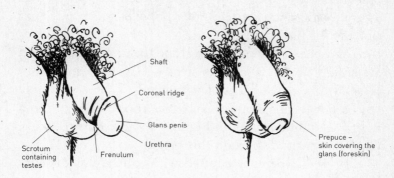

Shaft

Coronal ridge

Glans penis

Urethra

Scrotum
containing
testes

Frenulum

Prepuce –
skin covering the
glans (foreskin)

Figure 2.1: Anatomy of the penis: Non-erect, circumcised, and
uncircumcised

of lead pencils. Running through the bottom cylinder, so
that it's a little like a drinking straw, is the *urethra*, the tube
through which urine and sperm pass.

These cylinders of tissue are firmly held together by a
wrap of tissue called *Buck's fascia*. Buck's fascia is sort of
like industrial strength Glad Wrap and is important to the
functioning of the penis, as we'll discuss later.

The upper cylinders are each called *corpus cavernosum*
(plural *corpora cavernosa*). These are spongy tissue similar to a
bath sponge with spaces in between like a Swiss cheese.
Each of these cylinders is supplied by its own artery, and
this good blood supply assures a man's ability to have an
erection—when the sponges fill with blood, he's up. Putting
the lead in the pencil, you could say. More about this later.

The lower cylinder is called the *corpus spongiosum*. As we
mentioned, this contains the urethra, or tube through

which urine and sperm and seminal fluid pass (though not at the same time). It also contains two arteries that provide the blood supply.

The veins of the penis run along the upper surface and are readily visible when it is erect—they also can be felt, like the veins in the backs of your hands. The nerve supply to the penis runs along this surface too, breaking into a network of fine nerves and ensuring the exquisite sensations experienced through this organ.

The whole penis is covered with loose folds of skin. This skin becomes taut and deepens in color as the penis engorges with blood and rises. This color change is quite normal and not a cause for alarm; some old Chinese texts describe it prettily as "the blushing of the jade stem."

If a man has not been circumcised, he will have a hood-like fold of skin concealing the *head* or *glans* of the penis. This fold of skin is called the *foreskin*, and tends to be shorter in light-skinned races and longer amongst black men and those of Middle Eastern origin. In a man who has been circumcised, this skin has been removed and the glans will be obvious. The glans is a smooth bulbous cap of flesh at the end of the penis. Its skin is velvety and slightly darker than the shaft. The glans has a small vertical slit in it—this is the urethral opening, for the passage of urine and sperm. The foreskin, or hood of skin in an uncircumcised man, will retract, exposing the glans, when the penis becomes erect (see Figure 2.1 again for these various differences). In small boys who have not been circumcised, the foreskin may adhere to the glans—this is a variant of normal and sorts itself out as the boy grows older.

The *testicles*, aka the "balls" or "crown jewels," include the two *testes*—one on each side—each with a long coiled tube called the *epididymis*. Each epididymis acts as a conveying tube to carry the sperm from the testes, where they are manufactured, to the collecting tubes that ultimately carry them to the penis and outward. Just to keep things interesting, this voyage to the penis is somewhat tortuous—the tubes pass upward into the body and behind the bladder through a gland called the *prostate* and then they join into the urethra which, as you'll remember, is the tube that carries urine from the bladder (see Figure 2.2).

As the tubes travel from the testes to the space behind the bladder, they become known as the *vas deferens* (plural *vasa deferentia*)—this is where the term "vasectomy" comes from. The vas plus its nerve and blood supply, and the tissues surrounding it, form on each side the *spermatic cord*, which helps suspend the testis in the scrotum (see below).

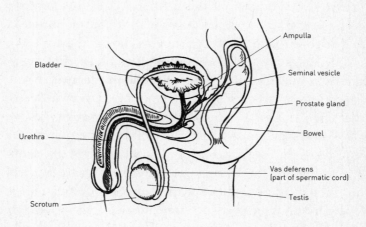

Figure 2.2: Functioning of the penis

Just before it enters the space behind the bladder, the vas opens out to form an individual sperm bank or collection center—the *ampulla*—where the sperm hang out until the call to fire comes through. Close to the ampulla, on either side, is a structure called the *seminal vesicle*, which produces *seminal fluid* (semen) which is added to the sperm. Seminal fluid plus sperm form the ejaculate produced at the climax of sexual intercourse. The ampulla and the seminal vesicle on each side join together, and the resultant single tube is called the *common ejaculatory duct* until it empties into the urethra.

In structure, the seminal vesicles are actually blind tubes coiled back on themselves—kinky, you might say. Each one can hold up to a full teaspoon of fluid. They are like a mountaineer's hut for the traveling sperm—a place to wait and get some energy in the form of fructose, a sugar that is produced in the seminal vesicles to help power the sperm. Also produced here is a fluorescent green coating on the sperm, the medical purpose of which is not clear (maybe so the egg can recognize it in the dark?).

The testes are veritable powerhouses of sperm manufacture. If only General Motors were so productive! If you looked under a microscope, you would find that the testis (the singular term) is made up of three main types of cells—one type consists of cells that become sperm (or, more correctly, "spermatozoa"). The second type make lots of nutrients for the spermatozoa to sustain them on their trip through all these tubes to their ultimate destination—hopefully (on their part) up some nice receptive vagina to fertilize a horny egg. Rather like the wolf's packed lunch until he meets Little Red Riding Hood. The final type of cell makes *testosterone*, the hormone responsible for a man's sex drive, as well as lots of other things, like his beard, acne, heavy muscles, and so forth.

The "balls" hang together in the loose bag of skin known as the *scrotum* or "ballbag" and beneath the skin is a thin layer of muscle called the *dartos*. The dartos is smooth muscle, which means it contracts in response to certain stimuli rather than by a conscious decision made in the brain. When the dartos contracts—in response to cold, sexual stimulation or for some other reason—the scrotum shrinks and its skin shrivels up like a dried prune.

The *prostate gland* is a structure about the size and shape of a chestnut that lies behind and below the bladder. The upper part of the urethra runs through the prostate from the bladder into the penis. Each of the common ejaculatory ducts also opens into this part of the urethra (see Figure 2.2). This is how sperm and seminal fluid get into the urethra, whereas urine obviously comes in from higher up, from the bladder.

The prostate gland has a large number of tiny ducts or openings from the gland into the urethra. Secretions from the gland become part of the seminal fluid or ejaculate as well. Although we will mention the prostate from time to time, we are confining this book to the penis, testes, and related structures. There are some good books available about the prostate—see Appendix 3 for more details.

Just as men's other physical features vary greatly, there is also great variation when it comes to Dick, in shape, color, and size. (OK, OK, we've written you a whole chapter on size, and we will tell you here that the human penis is the largest of any primate's.) There are also a number of benign conditions that may affect the appearance of Dick, which we'll tell you about in Chapter 13.

Dick has long been the subject of decoration. In New Guinea, elaborate penis sheaths, both straight and kinky, are created from gourds and are highly prized. Dick is sometimes tattooed in many societies, including our own, though in others—for example, in Polynesia—elaborate tattoos elsewhere on the body stop short of Dick. Certain societies who practice extensive body painting, for example in parts of Central Africa, always incorporate Dick into the color scheme. In modern life, Dick is generally, in his flaccid, placid state, tucked into jocks or boxers or allowed to swing free beneath kilt or sarong. Fashionable London tailors still ask their gentlemen clients which side they "dress," so that a little more fabric can be allowed for Dick's comfort. In Regency times, trendy young London men had metal rings inserted into their foreskins to anchor their equipment to their tight-fitting trousers so as not to spoil the line—today such rings are more a fashion statement.

It all helps to keep life interesting . . .

PHYSIOLOGY: THE UPS AND DOWNS OF A MOBILE ORGAN

3

Most men spend a fair bit of time thinking about their penises, we believe, but many of them have very little idea how the red hot poker actually works. When we talk about the physiology or function of the penis and its append-ages, we need to talk about urination, making sperm, performance of the sex act, and the production of male hormones. It's a good thing that a man doesn't have to think about the "how to" all the time!

The urge to pee begins in the bladder, which after infancy holds increasing amounts by keeping the muscle around the opening into the urethra firmly closed. As it approaches full capacity, signals are sent from the bladder via the nerves in the pelvis to the spinal cord. These signals generate a trigger back via the nerves to the bladder, causing the bladder to contract and the muscle—called a "sphincter"—leading to the urethra to relax, allowing the flow of urine through the urethra and out. These signals can be overridden by voluntary messages to the bladder from the brain until a suitable time and place for taking a leak is found. When the time is right, the voluntary messages are withdrawn and the bladder contracts and empties.

Gravity also plays a part in this process. Gravity, and the length and position of the male urethra, in contrast to the female, mean that urination in the male usually takes place standing up, whereas females squat or sit. So peeing in males is a much more visible, and hence competitive, occupation, leading to contests to see who can pee farthest in the snow or into the river—and not just amongst eight-year-olds!

Making sperm starts in puberty, roughly at the age of thirteen. It happens in the *seminiferous tubules*, which are serpentine coiled tubules in the testes containing specialized cells. When these cells are influenced by the male sex hormones, they enlarge, divide, and become *spermatocytes*, with a characteristic head, neck, body, and tail (see Figure 3.1). Each spermatocyte contains twenty-three chromosomes, half of the genetic information that is in each human cell. The spermatocytes mature and go through various changes to become fully fledged spermatozoa (sperm); this maturation process takes around sixty-four days, but sperm are continually being manufactured so at any time in the testis there are sperm at all stages of production. When the mature sperm fertilizes an egg, which also contains twenty-three chromosomes, the resultant embryo will have the full complement of forty-six chromosomes, with half from each parent.

After formation, these spermatocytes enter the epididymis on the same side (see Figure 2.2). They then make their way into the vas deferens and travel as far as the ampulla where they wait (patiently or impatiently) for ejaculation. Close to the ampullae, the seminal vesicles produce and store seminal fluid ready to add to the sperm. Both the sperm and the seminal fluid are channeled into an ejaculatory duct which, as we've seen, traverses the prostate gland to empty into the urethra. This whole process is constantly ongoing, but can be speeded by increased sexual demand.

So what's the point of the semen? To help the sperm in their swim. These little fellows don't wash through without some moisture. The fluid from the seminal vesicles comprises about 60 percent of the semen, but contributions are also made by fluid from the vas deferens and the prostate, and from mucous secretions in the urethra (see Figure 2.2).

The performance of the sex act has four physiological stages (see Figure 3.2). The first is *stimulation*. This is commonly initiated by emotional, visual, auditory, or even olfactory (smell) stimuli, all passing via the spinal cord to the nerves of the pelvis and then to the penis. Obviously the stimulus can be direct physical touch as well; in this respect, the glans or head of the penis is exquisitely sensitive, but messages still have to pass from the penis to the spinal cord and back again to be effective.

The second stage is *erection*, and this is the direct result of stimulation. Erection occurs when involuntary nerve impulses from the spinal cord cause the arteries in the penis to fill the spongy tissue cylinders with blood—similar to a garden hose that's filled with water when you turn on the tap. Buck's fascia acts like the rubber of the hose, holding everything firm. The arteries and smaller blood vessels have walls of smooth muscle that dilates, or opens out, so blood can enter quickly. This engorges the penis and causes it to harden, elongate, and rise at an angle to the belly. At the same time, the walls of the veins of the penis, which are quite thin, are held firmly together by the pressure of blood

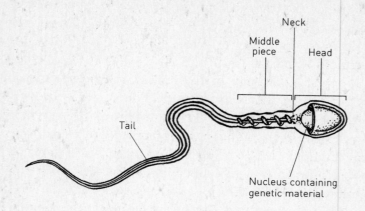

Neck

Middle
piece   Head

Tail

Nucleus containing
genetic material

Figure 3.1: Sperm structure

in the arteries and the spongy tissue. This prevents the
passage of blood back into the body from the penis, which
would cause it to flop too soon. During the process of
erection, more blood is coming into the penis than is going
out. It's worth noting here that getting a hard-on is something over which a man has little voluntary control; it's an
automatic response if the stimulation is there and the
nerves are working. (We believe it was St. Augustine who
first described Dick as having a mind of his own!)

Simultaneously, the third stage, *lubrication*, occurs. The
same spinal nerve impulses that are triggering erection
cause many little glands in the urethra to secrete mucus.
This may bead out and form a dew on the head of the
penis. While this is happening, there are changes occurring
in the rest of the body, with an increase in blood pressure,
pulse rate, and respiratory rate.

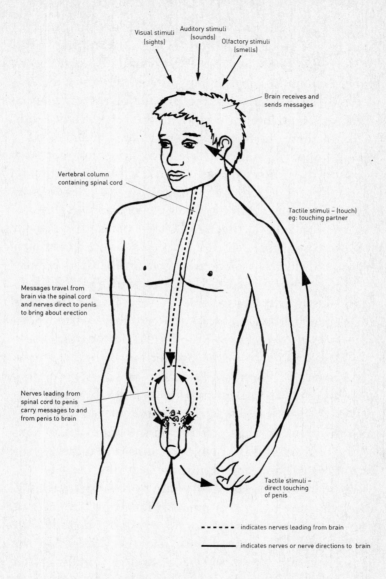

Visual stimuli (sights)

Auditory stimuli (sounds)

Olfactory stimuli (smells)

Brain receives and sends messages

Vertebral column containing spinal cord

Tactile stimuli – (touch) eg: touching partner

Messages travel from brain via the spinal cord and nerves direct to penis to bring about erection

Nerves leading from spinal cord to penis carry messages to and from penis to brain

Tactile stimuli – direct touching of penis

- - - - - indicates nerves leading from brain

——— indicates nerves or nerve directions to brain

Figure 3.2: The physiological mechanism of erection

Thrusting and *ejaculation* constitute the final stage. Stimulation of nerve endings on the skin and inside the penis transmit impulses to the spinal cord. In return, nerve impulses from the spinal cord trigger contractions of the epididymis, vas deferens, and the ampulla of the vas to eject sperm and fluid into the urethra. This mixes with the fluids secreted there, forming the semen, or ejaculate—also called spunk, come, cream, love-juice, jizz, cum, seed, and probably many other things. The filling of the urethra, in turn, triggers a reflex in the spinal cord, leading to rhythmic impulses sending waves of contractions through the smooth muscle that "milk" the penis and cause a forceful eruption of semen. This is ejaculation, also known as orgasm, climax, or "coming." Back in the third century AD, a Greek physician called Galen summed up the whole thing neatly when he wrote: "A very great pleasure is coupled with the exercise of the generative parts, and a raging desire precedes their use." That's for sure . . .

During ejaculation, the opening into the bladder is kept closed by contractions in the muscle surrounding it—this stops sperm entering the bladder. Ejaculation is followed by a decrease in the amount of blood coming into the penis and less pressure on the walls of the veins so the penis is emptied of blood, flops, and returns to its non-erect size and state. Until the next time . . .

Incidentally, semen doesn't have to have sperm in it—men who have had vasectomies, or men who have various conditions that prevent sperm production, still have perfectly good orgasms, with just the fluid from the seminal vesicles, prostate gland, and the urethra itself being ejaculated.

As we've said, the testes, as well as manufacturing sperm,

are the major production sites for male hormones. (One medical term for the testis is an "orchid"—removal of one of these exotic blooms is an orchidectomy, which we'll discuss later.) Testosterone is by far the most potent and abundant of the male hormones and will be the primary focus of our discussion.

Testosterone is formed in the testes by the *interstitial cells of Leydig*. A rather poetic name, don't you think? These cells are numerous in the newborn male and in men after puberty, but not in between. They secrete large amounts of testosterone. Interestingly, all testosterone is manufactured from the raw material of cholesterol. So you see, cholesterol is not all bad.

In the developing fetus, testosterone determines the development of the obvious sexual characteristics of the male baby—the penis and scrotum—as well as bringing about development of the prostate gland, seminal vesicles, and male genital duct. It also stimulates the descent of the testes into the scrotum and suppresses development of female sexual characteristics in the male baby.

At puberty, testosterone causes the penis, testes, and scrotum to enlarge. It also stimulates the growth of body hair in a diamond shape over the genital area and lower abdomen, the growth of hair in the armpits and on the chest, and generally makes body hair elsewhere thicker and more profuse. Ironically, it also contributes to male pattern baldness!

Testosterone causes the voice to deepen and the skin to thicken and to become oilier because of increased secretion from the sebaceous glands. This is the cause of that scourge of adolescence—acne. For most, the skin later adapts and acne ceases to be a problem. Another

21

effect is the bulking of muscle mass, leading to the typical male physique. Testosterone also has a building effect on bone, and boys' bones become denser and grow quickly in puberty. We see this as the famed "growth spurt."

Less talked about, but just as real, is the effect testosterone has on a man's sense of well-being. In recent years, it has been realized that the sex hormones act as powerful neurotransmitters in the brain, although we still have much to learn. Testosterone increases a man's basal metabolic rate and hence his energy level; if his testosterone levels are low, his energy level will be affected, as well as his libido. We'll tell you more about testosterone and other androgens (male hormones) in Chapter 4.

Before finishing our discussion of normal functioning, we'll just mention the subject of "nocturnal penile tumescence"—basically, erections occurring during sleep. This is a normal physiological event for all males from infancy to old age. In the healthy adult male, between two and five erections, each lasting for 25–35 minutes (yes, they've been intensively studied by scientists) and together accounting for up to 40 percent of sleep time, will occur each night. With advancing age, the number and duration of nighttime erections decreases. The "morning erection" many men observe (and often act upon!) is really a nighttime erection occurring just prior to waking and not, as is commonly supposed, due to a full bladder. It may, of course, be enhanced by a man finding his interested sexual partner lying beside him.

Most nighttime erections subside without the emission of semen. Around puberty though, and in the teenage years, nocturnal emissions frequently occur, and are completely normal.

HORMONES: "IT'S IN HIS BLOOD" 4

Expressions like "Ah, he's all hormones," or "it's just his hormones" are common, but what really are these hormones? A hormone is a messenger, a chemical substance that is produced in a gland in one part of the body and then carried by the blood to bring about effects in other parts of the body. It may also produce effects in the organ that makes it. Here we are talking about the male sex hormones and the pituitary hormones that regulate them.

The male sex hormones are called *androgens*. There are a number of them, but the major player is testosterone, (which we've already mentioned) produced in the testes in specialized cells called the Leydig cells. As we noted, cholesterol is the basic raw material for testosterone, as well as for all the steroid hormones, which includes all the androgens. We'll talk a little more about a couple of the others later in this chapter.

The output of testosterone by the Leydig cells is regulated by a feedback loop with the *pituitary gland*, which is a small gland in the brain, situated roughly behind the eyes (in both males and females). This, in turn, is directed by the *hypothalamus,* another brain area in very close proximity. Communication between these three is done via several different hormones conveying messages. The hypothalamus releases *gonadotrophin releasing hormone* (GnRH for short) and this tells the pituitary to release *luteinising hormone* (LH) which in turn stimulates the Leydig cells to produce testosterone. In return, the level of circulating testosterone signals the hypothalamus to turn off or decrease GnRH production until the testosterone levels fall or level out. This is like the boss taking a coffee break when the road gang is working and doing its job, but rising to his feet and yelling when he notices somebody slacking off. We have also provided a simplified diagram for you (see Figure 4.1).

What are the functions of the androgens? The first noticeable effect of testosterone is to cause the testes to descend into the scrotal sac, usually during the last couple of months of intra-uterine life. Testosterone is produced by the male foetus quite early on. Later, the increase in testosterone production at puberty causes the body changes associated with puberty—we'll talk about this in detail later on in this chapter.

Testosterone affects the distribution of hair on a man, causing the diamond-shaped fan of hair in the pubic area up to the navel, hair on the chest and sometimes back, and yes, contributes to the sparseness of hair up top! Baldness is attributable to a combination of genetic factors (just like your Dad's) and higher levels of androgens.

Male skin is thicker and typically oilier than that of females—this, too, is due to androgen production. Jim suffered with very oily skin and a lot of acne from age fourteen on—he also began to lose his hair at age

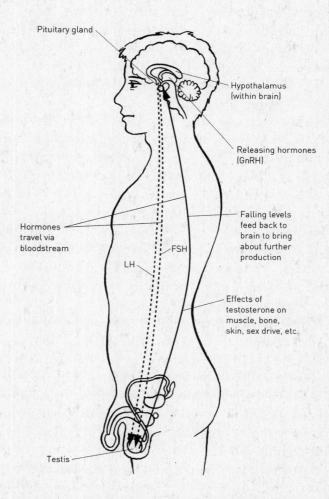

Figure 4.1: The hypothalamic–pituitary–testicular axis and hormonal pathways

twenty-five and was bald by thirty. His wife Marilyn was fond of rubbing his pate and telling everyone that he was the sexiest man she'd ever met! (Certainly there is some evidence that men who lose their hair early have higher levels of testosterone than others—though still within the normal range—and testosterone as we shall see is essential for male sex drive, so Marilyn may well be right.)

We all know that men have deeper voices than women—testosterone, again!

Testosterone is vitally important for muscle development. It is what initially triggers the typical male bulkiness of muscle mass and this is why androgens are being abused by athletes and bodybuilders. Unfortunately, the doses used are often dangerously high and the quality of the drug may make it unfit for human consumption.

Bones benefit from testosterone as well, and testosterone is necessary for normal bone growth and strength in men. Indeed, some women are given testosterone, in small doses, as a supplement after menopause when they show bone loss.

Metabolic rate is affected by testosterone—it speeds up all the basic activities and processes of the body's cells. The blood volume is also increased, as is the number of red blood cells. These effects may also be sought by athletes and bodybuilders, because they enhance athletic performance. Keep in mind that this is illegal and banned by various sports organizations for good reason: it is not a healthy thing to do.

Testosterone and the other androgens also have a mild effect on the balance of water and salts in the body. Under normal circumstances, this is insignificant compared with the effects of the hormones produced by the adrenal gland, but if you abuse androgens, normal may be turned on its head and these effects could be harmful. Yes, testosterone can be prescribed in a therapeutic manner, but this is only after blood levels have been checked and found to be low on at least two samples.

Last but not least, as we've already mentioned, testosterone gets the blue ribbon for keeping men sexually interested and motivated. Men with low testosterone, for whatever reason, typically have a low sex drive.

However, testosterone production is not the be all and end all—you still wouldn't produce sperm unless the pituitary gland put out *follicle stimulating hormone* (FSH), which supports the maturation of sperm in the testes. As you can see, managing the operations of the testes is an exquisitely organized process as complex as air traffic control.

At puberty, some unknown signal gears up the hypothalamus to secrete GnRH in a pulsatile pattern that stimulates the pituitary to release LH and FSH. Why and how it starts to do this some time between the ages of nine and fourteen in most boys is one of life's mysteries. But it does. We then see a recognizable pattern of development—the pubertal milestones. These are commonly referred to as the *Tanner stages* of adolescent development (see Table 4.1).

Boys often have concerns because they may be developing at different rates than their friends—obviously, if the age at which this all begins ranges from nine to fourteen, you will have boys in the same class at school at various stages of the process. This is quite normal and the average ages given on page 28 are just that—average. Boys should also be assured that the breast development they may see will not be with them all their lives—when the

Table 4.1: Pubertal milestones

Stage	Genitals	Growth in height	Pubic hair	Body signs
One	Childlike	2–2.5 in/yr	No	
Two	Scrotum thins and reddens [ave 11.9 yr] testes 1–1.3 in	2–2.5 in/yr	Scanty, darker hair around base of penis	Body lean
Three	Penis grows in length [ave 13.2 yr] testes 1.3–1.6 in	2.75–3 in/yr	Thicker, curly hair over mons pubis	Breast enlargement [ave 13.2 yr] Voice breaks [13.5 yr]
Four	Darkening of scrotum, growth of penis and glans testes 1.6–1.8 in	3–3.9 in/yr	Coarse, thick, curly hair but not yet on inner thighs	Armpit hair [14 yr] Voice deepens [14.2 yr] Acne [14.3 yr]
Five	Adult penis and glans [ave 15.1 yr] Testes >1.8 in	Levels off and stops	Adult type and spread to inner thighs	Beard growth [14.9 yr] Muscle mass increasing

surge of development calms down, the breasts naturally regress, leaving our hero with his manly form.

Jake and Lou are good examples. Jake was the tallest kid in class by the time he was fourteen. He had begun developing when he was nine and a half and by age fourteen was burly and had a baritone voice that only cracked when he was reciting in front of the class. His best friend Lou, on the other hand, still looked like a little kid at fourteen. He was only just beginning to have the first few hairs around his weenie and had yet to see a zit. By age eighteen, though, Lou was a good six inches taller than Jake and all their other attributes were on par.

If your child shows no sign of development by fourteen or fifteen, just have your doctor check him. Developmental disorders are not very common, but they do occur. If he is one of the early bloomers, remember that his emotional development has not kept pace and he is still a child—so have patience.

What about the other end of the spectrum? Is there a male equivalent to menopause? Strictly speaking, no. Male hormone output does decline with age, but it is a slow and gradual thing, not like the dramatic time that women may go through. And, as many have noted, men can and do father children at very advanced ages. This is not true for women.

Some doctors say that there exists an androgen deficiency syndrome, especially as men age. John Morley, M.D., developed a questionnaire that correlates symptoms with low testosterone levels (see Table 4.2).

If you answer three or more of these questions positively, then your serum testosterone should be checked, according to some geriatrics experts. (We know what you're saying: lots of people of all ages, male and female, would probably answer yes to at least three of these . . .) If low, these experts would supplement you with testosterone. This is controversial, and we still don't have enough information to indicate whether androgen replacement is in the same category as female hormone replacement.

Table 4.2: Correlation of symptoms with low testosterone

1 Do you have a decrease in sex drive?
2 Do you have lack of energy?
3 Do you have a decrease in strength or endurance?
4 Have you lost height?
5 Do you enjoy life less?
6 Are you sad and/or grumpy?
7 Are your erections weaker?
8 Do you feel your emotions less?
9 Do you fall asleep after dinner?
10 Has your work performance deteriorated?

There *are* risks to androgen supplementation, and these must be acknowledged. First, as our colleague Dr. Cohen cautions, if you are brewing a little prostatic cancer, adding additional testosterone to your system may be like throwing kerosene on a fire. Also, oral testosterone endangers your liver; for this reason, most doctors do not prescribe it. It is available by injection or transdermally (through the skin) as a patch or gel.

Testosterone does increase muscle mass and may seem tempting to men who have lost lean mass with aging. It is not yet known whether testosterone supplementation helps to reverse the decrease in bone mass that is natural to aging men. And if it does reverse bone loss, does it also reduce fractures? The jury is still out.

Some argue that androgen supplementation will protect men against Alzheimer's. Maybe . . . we just don't have the studies to support this yet.

Besides liver toxicity and possible acceleration of prostate cancer, androgens can cause water retention, and this may pose an increased risk for men with high blood pressure or heart disease. It may also worsen sleep apnea; it is thought that this happens by causing a thickening of the tissues at the back of the throat.

Probably the biggest controversy raging is about the effect of androgens on blood fats. There are conflicting studies—some showing that HDL (good cholesterol) is reduced by supplementing with androgens, some showing no effect, and some actually indicating a beneficial effect. For now, it is probably best to be cautious and discuss all of this with a trusted doctor who knows you and your particular situation and risks. And if you should at any point be prescribed supplemental androgens, be sure that you are monitored at least every six months.

As mentioned, oral testosterone is not a great idea. Injectable testosterone has been used for decades and is the least expensive route of administration. In recent years, testosterone patches have come on the market and offer a closer match to the physiological pattern of testosterone release, with peaks early in the day and a diminution toward evening.

Up until now, we've pretty much spoken of androgens and testosterone interchangeably. There are, however, a couple of other androgens worthy of some mention, mostly because they are being sold and used as "dietary supplements" and are readily available over the Internet and, at least in the United States, in health food stores. These are *DHEA* and *pregnenolone*. These are weaker androgens than testosterone and are precursors in the chain of synthesis from cholesterol. Although weaker, they can have many of the same effects as testosterone and presumably the same ill-effects. In fact, we don't know enough about the results of using these pharmacologically. Studies are under way, and there are some diverse and hopeful signs (e.g. that DHEA may increase bone mass in older women), but it is premature as yet to make any ethical claims about these androgens.

Another interesting androgen is *dihydrotestosterone*, the metabolite of testosterone that is active in the cells. It is at least theorized that topical drugs that block dihydrotestosterone in the scalp cells will allow a rejuvenation of hair growth. In fact, a couple of preparations based on this are now on the market.

Saeed had been buying an expensive drug to grow a little more fuzz on his bald pate. He was delighted when his chemist told him about a cream he could rub in and that it would cost him just a fraction of the current drug. So far, Saeed hasn't seen much difference . . .

Your hormonal system is a very finely tuned mechanism. As you can see, it determines your sexual characteristics and thereby your presentation to the world. Our advice to every man would be to take care not to disturb this fine balance by monkeying with illicit androgens.

HYGIENE: LET'S KEEP IT CLEAN . . . 5

The message in this chapter is brief and to the point: A clean pecker is a healthy pecker. And a healthy pecker makes for a happy cocksman.

Smegma is a cheesy substance that forms under the foreskin of uncircumcised men. It is composed of natural skin lubricants, exfoliated skin cells, and the bacteria that live harmoniously on all our skins. In and of itself, smegma is not unclean—it is a natural body by-product. However, when it is allowed to accumulate through lack of washing, it provides a fertile breeding ground for bacteria and viruses and contributes to inflammation. It will also become malodorous and not contribute to one's charm. A simple daily wash with water and a mild soap takes care of any potential problems here.

Adam has two young sons and enjoys bathing them each night. When each boy reached three years of age, Adam started showing them how to gently pull back their foreskins and wash their tiny sticks well themselves. It may be a game at this point, but will be a good habit for these boys for the rest of their lives.

In many areas of our lives, we need to take protective measures to ensure our safety and health. This is true in our sexual lives as well, and the cocksman who goes into action without a sheath—rubber, condom, or whatever you wish to call them—is a very foolhardy man. Yes, there may be a slight difference in sensation, but you do climax and you do it with the peace of mind that you won't be trading a minute's fun for a major illness. Much more about this later in our chapter on condoms.

Hygiea was the Greek goddess of health and talking of hygiene leads naturally to the consideration of health measures beyond cleanliness. Dick doesn't function well if the rest of your body is not well nourished, free of toxins, and rested. As you will see from stories later in this book, excessive alcohol can really impair Dick's ability to perform, even if it heightens the desire to do so.

As with every other part of your body, your little buddy works best when the rest of you does, so improving nutrition never hurts. A diet high in fruits, vegetables, and high-quality protein, including fish and lean meats, is ideal. (For more details see Chapter 22.) If you have familial tendencies toward diabetes or heart disease, it is especially important to eat healthily and keep your weight within 10 percent of the optimum. This is best based on a measurement of your body mass index and not just straight weight. Many gyms and doctors' offices can measure this for you, and bathroom scales that read this measurement are now available.

Exercise has been shown to be valuable for circulatory health, and good circulation is needed for old Dick to get it up. You don't need to be a jock, but don't be a couch potato either.

Finally, take care to protect the family gems from injury—athletic cups are not just for adolescents in competitive sports. It is not a bad idea to wear them whenever you play casual sports or use power tools. Accidents are always a surprise, so prevention is never frivolous—see some salutary anecdotes and our words of advice in Chapter 17.

6   SIZE: DOES IT MATTER?

Recent email messages:

Increase your penis size by 1 ... 2 ... 3 inches or more in just a few short weeks!

Former Viagra pharmacist has now created a revolutionary herbal pill that is guaranteed to increase your penis size by 1 inch ... 2 inches ... 3 inches ... or more in just a few short weeks!

This amazing new product works by simply taking two pills every day ... it will make your penis grow in both length and thickness by a whopping 25 percent, guaranteed!

Click here for details

In a few years, we will have a lot of people running around with huge breasts and long dicks who won't remember what to do with them (Tommer001).

2:52 P.M. Police were called to the scene of a six-foot snow sculpture in the shape of a male sexual organ ... (Amherst, MA police blotter).

There is a myth that bigger is better in regard to penises. This is analogous to "blondes have more fun" or "you can never be too thin or too rich." In all cases, this refers to success, especially in the bedroom. Bigger equates with more powerful, more forceful, more masculine and being better in the sack. But this, we believe, is a "phallusy."

A quick surf of the Internet will demonstrate the hidden (or not so hidden) desire of many men to have a larger penis. Literally thousands of results come up (forgive us!) when you type "penis" into your search bar, and more than 99 percent of these are advertisements similar to the one quoted above.

The average size of the erect penis, according to numerous independent investigators, is about five and a half inches and this varies much less than the size of flaccid penises. (No, in case you're wondering, it is not predicted by the size of a man's nose or feet or any other obvious clues.) In contrast, the penis of a gorilla is only two inches long. At the other extremes are the penises of pigs, which are almost eighteen inches long, and those of humpback whales, coming in at almost ten feet! Despite wide interest in "twelve-inch clubs," the longest recorded human penis actually comes in at a little longer, 12.99 inches (no, we're *not* telling you who or where).

Our research has shown that interest in size occurs in many parts of the globe, from Japan to the Caribbean. In the town of Komaki, Central Japan, an ancient Shinto fertility rite is conducted regularly in which a six and a half foot-high wooden phallus is paraded through town, while women hold mini-models of the symbol and stroke and kiss the big tickler for good luck. In the West Indies, cricketer Joel Garner, who stood over seven feet in his socks, was once asked by a bold reporter if the size of his old fellow was in proportion to his height. "No, man," was the response. "If dat was the case I'd be sixteen feet tall." And so it goes . . .

In the Middle Ages in Europe, men of fashion wore long pointed shoes to try to indicate to the ladies that they were especially well-endowed beneath their codpieces. Church and state authorities tried in vain to forbid the wearing of these early crotch enhancers. Some men emphasized the message by wearing bells on their toes. A few guys who thought they were God's gift had shoes so long the toes were tied to the owners' belts, so they could walk. Whether shaft length actually matched shoe length is not recorded . . .

Codpieces too were more about size than keeping out chills. They were originally prescribed by church authorities who thought men's jackets were becoming too short. But the codpieces got bigger and more ostentatious, some men covered them with jewels (yes, we know that expression), others kept their wallets there, and there was even a device that could attach a flagpole to your codpiece (giving new meaning to "raising the flag"). Certainly a good codpiece could catch a lady's eye, but it may have promised more than it could deliver.

The size of the erect penis is designed to get the job done, and the job in question is to impregnate the woman and assure continuity of the species. In the *Kama Sutra,* one of the oldest sex manuals, men are divided into three classes based on penis size. (We're not told who decided this, or who did the classifying!) They are called the Hare, the Bull, and the Horse.

The Hare is not longer than five inches in the erect state and has a sweet semen. Its owner is calm and depicted as short and compact. The Bull is not longer than seven inches and its owner is always hot to trot. He is described physically as having a high forehead, large eyes, and robust health. The Horse is a whopping ten inches with copious salty semen. However, its owner is described as tall and large, slow and lazy, with only sporadic interest in sex.

The same text classifies women's vaginas into three categories based on size and claims that the best sex is when the size of the penis and that of the vagina are similar. But in fact the vagina is an expansile organ designed to adapt itself around the entering member. When a woman first starts to have intercourse, there may be some pain and bleeding because the hymen, the ring of tissue around the vaginal opening, has been torn or stretched and has to heal, which can take a number of days. Using a lubricant like KY jelly or Astroglide (or even baby oil) may help here. But beyond the hymen the vagina itself consists of stretchy tissue that molds around the penis, the two becoming basically complementary in size to each other. After childbirth, the vagina does not always return to its original degree of elasticity. However, it will still mold to fit the erect penis, and pelvic floor exercises (Kegel's) done regularly will help to restore muscle strength and vaginal tone.

The size of a man's equipment has little to do with how good a lover he is; but how he uses it does. The writer Balzac said that "the love-making of many men resembles a gorilla trying to play a violin." But he was living in the nineteenth century when this subject was not discussed in polite society and women often thought of sex as something they had to put up with to stay married. In the twenty-first century, frank discussion between partners about sexual wants and satisfaction is widely accepted, in Western countries at least, as normal. A man who truly cares about his partner's responses and satisfaction and who gives her tenderness and time is a far better lover than a man with a slightly larger penis who mechanically goes through the sex manual motions, with little true concern for his partner. And woe betide the man with the truly large penis—he may find that his organ gives pain, rather than pleasure. Satisfying sex usually has little to do with the size of the conjoined organs but everything to do with the sensitivity of each partner to the other's needs and desires. It is not an athletic sport, but instead a manifestation of an intimate relationship.

As women, we may not be able to dispel completely the myth that a large penis signifies great sexual prowess, but we can be sensitive to our lovers' fears of inadequacy in this department.

A MAJOR HANDFUL: MASTURBATION 7

In the recent bestseller *The Royal Physician's Visit,* by Per Olav Enquist, we read that the mad young King Christian of Denmark was habituated to a secret vice. Testimony taken at the time attributed his melancholy, fits of passion, rages, and periods of profound apathy to this vice. It was a very well-known secret. It was stated that this vice was the cause of his dementia, weakened his physical constitution and paralyzed his will. The less timorous named this vice: masturbation. Did the fate of a small eighteenth-century Nordic country rise and fall on one palm and five fingers?

What is masturbation? One definition is sexual activity involving only one person; synonymous are self-stimulation, auto-eroticism, and self-pleasure. It usually means stimulating one's own genitals in such a way as to lead to sexual excitement and orgasm. Obviously a little more action is needed than a quick wash is likely to provide. Most commonly, a man will use his hands and fingers, but occasionally he will find pleasure from rubbing his penis with various objects. Shane liked a special piece of silk fabric. The original was from a dress

that belonged to a lover and the silk became part of a rich
sexual fantasy.

There is much evidence that masturbation is part of
almost every man's sex life. Dr. Alfred Kinsey, after inter-
viewing thousands of men, concluded in 1948 that 95
percent of them masturbated; in 1966, Masters and
Johnson put the proportion closer to 99 percent. An
informal online survey, reported on the Jackinworld Web
site, indicates that the greatest frequency of masturbation
is among eleven-year-olds, with frequency declining to
about five times weekly in men over thirty-five. We don't
know how far over thirty-five they polled . . .

There is now a fairly wide-reaching consensus among
health professionals that masturbation is something that
almost everyone practices and that it has a role to play in
maintaining the emotional and psychological health of
the individual. It is also pointed out that, for adolescents,
masturbation is a much safer sexual outlet than unprotected sexual intercourse, with its ramifications of STDs
and unwanted pregnancies and the emotional entangle-
ments that a teenager may be too immature to handle in
a healthy way. In spite of these views, masturbation can
still raise official eyebrows; in 1994 U.S. Surgeon General
Joycelyn Elders was asked to resign within hours of
publicly stating that "perhaps masturbation is something
that should be taught" in reference to public school health
education—an example of a policy of prudery, not
common sense.

What are the potential benefits of masturbating? First
of all, one is able to explore his (or her) own sexuality
without the inappropriate involvement of another person
(for example, fantasies about a big blonde with enormous

you-know-whats, when your main squeeze is a petite redhead). In addition, sexual release is a great remedy for generalized anxiety and can help promote relaxation. Many couples enjoy mutual masturbation as part of their sexual relationship: it does not cause pregnancy, nor does it transmit disease.

What are the arguments against masturbation? In Victorian times, doctors warned darkly that "the effects of masturbation were worse than those of most diseases—the frequent masturbator was pale, downcast, couldn't sleep and had damp, cold hands." Good Lord! Today there are no medical arguments against this practice, although you will still find religious objections, primarily from conservative religious practitioners. To quote Monty Python: "Every sperm is sacred; every sperm is great. If a sperm is wasted, God gets quite irate." The arguments proffered usually run along the lines that sex is for procreation alone and therefore masturbation, since it cannot result in pregnancy, is an unnatural act. The only natural act is sexual intercourse that can result in pregnancy; therefore, by this reasoning, practicing safe sex is also unnatural. Pope Paul VI in *Persona Humana* declared that "masturbation constitutes a grave moral disorder" and "even if it cannot be proved that Scripture condemns this sin by name, the tradition of the Church has rightly understood it to be condemned in the New Testament when the latter speaks of 'impurity,' 'unchasteness,' and other vices contrary to chastity and continence."

These are matters of faith and conscience; however, the widespread practice of masturbation would indicate that people who adhere to the belief that it is a vice and a sin still do it, but feel guilty about it. Which is a pity.

Max is a big, burly fellow who works a variety of jobs to support his one true love: music. Max shared a deep dark secret with his doctor one day—he "jerked off" about six times daily and was afraid that that was the true cause of his tummy cramps and constipation. He confessed that he used to do this even more often but was trying to control the urge. Our friend the doc was able to convince Max that his sexual habits had nothing to do with his tummy troubles—he was sensitive to the gluten in wheat products and his love of pasta and bread was the direct cause, not his relationship with his action man.

We are not religious authorities and we make no moral statements about masturbation. However, as doctors, we can say with certainty that you will not go blind, become demented, lose your hair, lose your ability to relate to other human beings, become psychotic or retarded in your physical growth, or lose your ability to be a productive member of society if you masturbate.

CIRCUMCISION: THE UNKINDEST CUT? 8

Circumcision is, by and large, surgery performed for social and cultural reasons—rarely for medical indications. In fact, the decision to circumcise an infant is almost always made without any medical opinion being asked for or expressed.

The practice of circumcision has been around for a very long time. Circumcision of male Jewish infants on the eighth day after birth is a rite accompanied by prescribed ceremonies and benedictions and the naming of the child; it represents part of Abraham's Covenant with God, who is said in Genesis to have told Abraham specifically that "ye shall circumcise the flesh of your foreskin." Circumcision has also been universally practiced amongst Muslim people, though at varying ages—often soon after birth, before puberty, or sometimes just before marriage if the man has converted. Traditional Muslim belief is that an uncircumcised man cannot enter heaven.

The same serious view of circumcision has been taken by people as widely separated as the Polynesians and the Masai of East Africa—the latter practice elaborate rituals associated with circumcision for boys between the ages of twelve and sixteen. Traditional Australian Aboriginal societies also used circumcision as a rite of passage for boys from childhood to adulthood. In all these societies the time-honored instrument for performing the procedure was a stone knife rather than a metal one, something that testifies to the antiquity of the practice.

The need for circumcision was disputed in the early Christian church (for those interested in an account of this, turn to Acts 15!), so it has never been a Christian religious requirement, nor has it been a Christian belief that this perceived male design defect must be corrected in order to enter the Pearly Gates. However, obviously a good many Christians have been circumcised, usually as infants.

What is involved in circumcision? Jennifer, who had grown up with three sisters and had never seen a little boy's penis, had no real concept of what circumcision meant. Her first-born was a boy and she agreed with her husband when he said: "Well, his daddy is circumcised so he should be, too." It was only later that the reality that little Georgie had had a surgical procedure done hit home for Jennifer. She was learning to change his nappies and bathe him and there was that little red-tipped willie, surrounded by Vaseline-coated gauze and looking so sore that she cried.

When we circumcise a baby, we cut off the loose tube of skin that slips up and down the shaft of the penis and covers the head or glans. The tube of skin slips back naturally when the penis is erect, but covers it in the flaccid state. There are many methods of doing this, but among the most common is slipping a metal or plastic bell-shaped instrument over the glans penis, under the foreskin (the part we are going to cut off), to protect the glans and then cutting the foreskin off along the edge provided by the bell. The latest guidelines from pediatric specialists state that adequate anesthesia should be provided. This is not how it has always been; it was routine to circumcise babies without any local anesthetic as recently as the 1980s, with the rationale that infants didn't experience pain in the same way as older children and adults and that the use of local anesthetic made the procedure a bit more technically difficult. Fortunately, we are more enlightened now and it is current policy to always use adequate anesthesia.

Why do parents choose to circumcise their sons? Pediatrician Dr. Jeffrey Tiemstra studied a large group of parents requesting circumcision for other than religious reasons—asked for their main reasons, 67 percent cited the ease of keeping the baby clean, 63 percent said that it was so much easier to be circumcised as a baby than as an adult if it had to be done, 41 percent cited possible medical benefits, and 37 percent said that the baby's father was circumcised and the baby should look like his daddy.

Are there really any medical benefits to circumcision? Traditionally, parents were told that the procedure reduced the risks of penile cancer, infant urinary infection, and, later, sexually transmitted diseases. In fact, these benefits are not medically compelling. It is true that urinary tract infection occurs more often in uncircumcised babies than in those who have been circumcised, but this must be understood in the context of an overall risk of less than 1 percent. It is doubtful that we would amputate a finger for a 1 percent risk of infection. Simple hygiene—gently retracting the foreskin and keeping the area clean with soap and water—will greatly reduce the chances of infection.

The overall risk of penile cancer is one in 100,000 men, another less-than-striking risk factor. Using this type of rationale, we should be doing mastectomies on all little girls to protect against breast cancer.

As far as STDs are concerned, it has been well demonstrated that behavioral factors have much more to do with one's risk of STD than any little appendage of skin.

Interestingly enough, in studies and in the experience of physicians who perform circumcisions, informing parents of these facts has little impact on their decision to circumcise, and often antagonizes parents. Those parents studied who chose not to circumcise their children stated that they thought the procedure unnecessary and painful.

Official policy is to honor the wishes of parents concerning circumcision and to ensure that it is done only on healthy infants and with adequate anesthesia. We should not, however, lose sight of the fact that it is unnecessary surgery performed on children who cannot give informed consent.

ADULT CIRCUMCISION

Adult circumcision is performed much less commonly than infant circumcision. It is more commonly done for medical reasons, such as phimosis, paraphimosis, recurrent balanitis, or posthitis.

What the **** *are* these, you say? *Phimosis* is a very tight foreskin that will not retract back over the glans of the penis. This may cause pain during erection or intercourse (and, of course, you can't have intercourse without an erection). *Paraphimosis* is a retracted foreskin that won't slip back over the glans. This causes a painful swelling of the glans and when this happens acutely—say, after a bee sting while pissing in the bush—paraphimosis can be a urological emergency because it can seriously interfere with the ability to urinate. Michele's most memorable case of paraphimosis was that of a small boy who peed on an electric fence—the electricity arced back and burnt his glans. *Balanitis* is inflammation or infection of the glans, and *posthitis* is an inflammation of the foreskin itself. None of these is very common—the most common is phimosis followed by paraphimosis.

As an adult, it is important that you understand the risks of circumcision before consenting to the procedure: these include bleeding, hematoma (a large bruise), infection, inadvertent damage to the glans, the taking of too much or too little foreskin, and cosmetically displeasing results. Obviously, too, parents should be aware of these risks before formally consenting to circumcision for their newborn sons. As far as adult circs are concerned, it must also be understood that the sensations of intercourse may be different from before, not as sharp, it has been said, and that erections may be painful in the post-op period and, in fact, may disrupt the stitches, so sex is a no-no at this time. Full recovery and return to sexual activity may take four to six weeks.

Local anesthetic, blocking sensation to the whole penis, is used in adults, and the operation is usually done as an outpatient. Aftercare involves loose briefs and, if desired, petrolatum gauze dressings.

Once in a while, a man may have social or cultural reasons for requesting circumcision. Jeremy wanted to marry the love of his life, Rachel, but her family would not consent unless he converted to Judaism. Jeremy converted and included a semi-ritual circumcision conducted by both a physician and a rabbi. (Our urologist colleague Dr. Arthur Cohen has helpfully informed us that ritual in this situation, rather than requiring full circumcision, can be served by a token surgical event—which he describes as "a prick on a prick." Thanks, Arthur!)

VASECTOMY: TYING THE KNOT 9

Tony and Maria and their two children, dog, and cat are a typical modern family. They all live together in the suburbs, in a brick house with a sizeable mortgage; he's a building inspector for the city and she works part-time in a library.

After Maria had her second child, Rosa, by cesarean three years ago, she developed a blood clot in her leg and lung. Fortunately this was quickly diagnosed and Maria started on anti-coagulant treatment. Her doc told her that this meant she would be wise not to have any more pregnancies and also said that she shouldn't take the Pill. "Don't worry," said Tony, "it's my turn to go and have surgery—after all, it's only a little cut."

The trouble is, Rosa's now enrolled in kindergarten and Tony still hasn't got those knots tied. A mate at work told him about his cousin's friend's friend, who couldn't get it up after having a vasectomy . . . and somebody else Tony knows had read an article linking vasectomy to heart attacks. Maria doesn't want any of these things to happen to Tony any more than he does, but she's been worried sick about accidentally getting pregnant again—they use condoms but she knows there's a failure rate with these. Now she's read the riot act—there's an appointment for Tony next week to at least go and talk to the doctor and get these questions answered.

As Tony himself admits, vasectomy—or male sterilization—is a relatively simple operation. You'll remember (from Chapter 2) the vas deferens, the tube that brings sperm from the testis to the penis—one vas on either side. The sperm then hang around until they are called upon, in the ampulla of the vas (see Figures 2.1 and 2.2).

When a vasectomy is done, the vas deferens are cut or clamped, as in Figure 9.1. This blocks the passage of the sperm from the testes to the urethra and therefore makes the ejaculated fluid sterile. Sperm production continues in the testes but the sperm are simply broken down and reabsorbed by the body with no unpleasant side-effects.

A vasectomy is very often done in a doctor's office, although some doctors may prefer to do it as an outpatient at their local hospital. The skin of the scrotum is numbed with a local anesthetic, one or two tiny cuts are made in the skin, and each vas is pulled out into a small loop. The arc of the loop is cut. The raw ends of the severed loop will then be stitched, tied, or burned closed (see Figure 9.1). This helps prevent their growing back together. Each vas deferens is then slipped back into the scrotum and the tiny incisions are sutured closed. The whole procedure takes only about twenty to thirty minutes.

Vasectomy, like tubal ligation in women, is a permanent method of birth control and a man must be clear in his own mind that he is at peace with this decision. He needs to consider how he would feel if he should lose his present partner, through death or divorce, or if one or more of his children were to die. It is hard to be certain how you might feel in these circumstances, but it is important to think about them before making a decision about what needs to be regarded as an irreversible procedure.

Yes, reversals are done—the two ends of the vas deferens can be joined up again, using microsurgery. But this doesn't mean that they will function as they used to— it's not just like fixing a broken water pipe. Also it seems that sometimes the sperm "trapped" in the testes may undergo changes so they are less effective at producing a pregnancy if a reversal is carried out. The pregnancy rate after reversal of vasectomy is around 40–70 percent, depending on how long it was since the vasectomy, the skill of the surgeon, and many other factors.

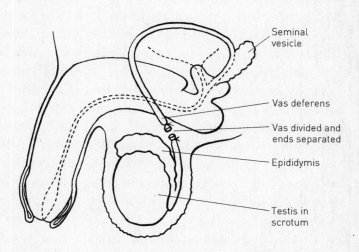

Seminal vesicle

Vas deferens

Vas divided and ends separated

Epididymis

Testis in scrotum

Figure 9.1: Vasectomy

Vasectomy is minor surgery and has fewer risks and complications than tubal ligation does in women. For a start, only local anaesthesia is needed, and the abdominal cavity does not need to be entered. The only likely complication of the procedure is some bruising—treated with ice-packs, firm support briefs, and tender sympathy from a loved one, this should soon ease.

Vasectomy is extremely effective as a contraceptive measure, but not quite 100 percent. Very occasionally, the ends of the vas can join spontaneously and sperm can get through to fertilize an egg. This happens in about 0.1 percent of men who have had a vasectomy.

Tony did finally get to the appointment with Dr. Cohen and in the waiting room he met David. David explained that he'd had the op four months previously and was here for the results of his final sperm count—after the vasectomy, sperm can still be present in the ampulla and two negative sperm counts are necessary before the man gets the "all clear." David explained that he and his wife Belinda had one lovely daughter, Tahlia, and Belinda had experienced a difficult birth. Though they both adored Tahlia, David and Belinda were adamant that they did not want more children and David had opted to get "fixed." Hesitating a bit, Tony then told David about his fears of not getting it up. David laughed: "No, mate," he said. "Just the opposite is what we've found, now that we're no longer worried about Belinda getting pregnant again. And once we get the word today, we can stop using condoms altogether."

Dr. Cohen confirmed this to Tony, explaining that erection and orgasm occur exactly as before vasectomy, except that the ejaculate no longer contains sperm. He also assured him that vasectomy had not been linked to heart disease in any way, and told him about a World Health Organization study that had found no connection between vasectomy and cancer of the prostate, or any other cancer. He cautioned Tony to be very sure about his decision, and sent him away to think about it.

The upshot was that two weeks later Tony had a vasectomy carried out in Dr. Cohen's office, with a very contented Maria waiting outside to drive him home. Four months later, they celebrated Tony's zero sperm count with a weekend without the kids, in the seaside resort where they'd spent their honeymoon.

10 USING YOUR JOYSTICK

It has never been intended that *Dick* should be a sex manual, but given that there are two basic uses for the penis, and sex is one of them, it is appropriate to at least raise the flag and salute the first and best form of entertainment in this chapter.

There exists today a certain ennui in regard to sex, thanks to the topic being somewhat overdone in the popular press. However, the act itself is by definition exciting.

Our far distant ancestors went about on all fours and knew only one sexual position—rear entry. As we began to walk in the erect posture, the opportunities to explore a variety of sexual positions arose and so did good old Dick. Presumably, the notions of romantic love and intimacy became entwined with sex after men and women faced each other while enjoying their coupling. This is conjecture, because our early forbears were more interested in doing it than writing about it.

There are many sex manuals, from the *Kama Sutra*, written about 2000 years ago and the ancient pillow books of Japan to more recent offerings (you will find a small list in the appendix). The Kama Sutra lists eighty-four positions, many of which require incredible flexibility and acrobatic ability. It also offers the very sensible advice: "Women being of a tender nature, want tender beginnings."

Foreplay is very important; the Dicktator is always ready to command, but a woman's maximal pleasure is dependent upon stimulation of her clitoris, using either the fingers, penis, or tongue. In the *Perfumed Garden*, translated by Sir Richard Burton, it compares the woman to the basil plant "which will not emit a warm scent unless rubbed with fingers." A woman's pleasure heightens her partner's pleasure, both emotionally and by the squeezing sensations of her contracting vagina on his penis. The joystick gives pleasure to both partners. The touch should be light and gentle and women should tell their partners how they like to be touched. One of the most common complaints women have is that Dick is too rough. Be gentle.

Variety is nice. Barbara has been married to Glen for ten years. She said that she has begun having less satisfaction in the sexual part of their marriage because "it's the same old thing: every Saturday night, we go out for dinner at the same place and go bowling with our friends, have a couple of drinks and then it's home and slam, bam, thank you m'am, in the same old missionary position with exactly three kisses and a little rub first." Variety doesn't mean that you have to take yoga lessons so you can do some of the more difficult positions . . . it does mean being a little more creative and perhaps consulting one of the time-honored sex manuals. You may laugh a lot as you try some of the new things, but, then, sex is supposed to be fun, isn't it?

There is no shame or abnormality in any sexual gratification between consenting adults who are respectful of each other as human beings, whether it's a straightforward roll in the hay or a 69 experiment, or any variation on the theme.

In the Middle Ages, guys wore shoes that had long pointed toes, colored pink and stuffed with wool and anything else handy to keep them bouncy and erect. Sometimes, they were even tethered by a cord to the knees. These toe extensions were supposedly representative of what was hidden under the guy's codpiece—the bigger and bouncier the toes, the bigger and bouncier the you-know-what. Today, tight jeans, Speedo swim suits, and athletic tights and shorts advertise in much the same manner.

Initiation into sex often takes the form of a group jerk off, with anywhere from two to five or six adolescents participating. They also exchange the bits and pieces of information that each has gleaned from friends, books, personal experience, and once in awhile, parents. Much of this information is short on accuracy, but gains veracity with repeating.

Rules for Sex

1. Remember there are a limited number of orifices in the body—Dick has tried all and some work better than others.
2. A clean Dick is happier than a smelly one.
3. Gently, gently goes it.
4. A rubber keeps Dick a happy fellow, with no serious regrets.
5. Ask first.
6. Be considerate of your partner—no one wants to feel like a receptacle.
7. If at first it doesn't work, relax and try again.
8. Alcohol and drugs are deflating influences.
9. Have fun!

11 SEX AFTER 50 . . . AND 60 . . . "IT'S STILL HAPPENING!"

Lionel (eighty) and Jean (seventy-eight) met in a retirement village and have finally decided to get married. They are walking hand-in-hand, like a couple of teenagers, down the street to the coffee shop. Suddenly, Lionel directs Jean into the pharmacy they are passing.

Lionel begins to question the person behind the counter: "Do you sell high blood pressure medicine? Diabetes medications?"

"Yes, certainly, sir."

"How about painkillers for arthritis?"

"Yes, all kinds."

"Viagra?" Lionel turns a little pink as he asks this.

"Of course."

"Do you carry the new medicines for Alzheimer's?"

"Indeed we do."

"How about supplies, like walkers, wheelchairs, walking sticks?"

"Yes, a full supply, all speeds and sizes."

Lionel turns to his new bride: "Well, Jean, I think
this is the place to register for wedding gifts."

With the growing number of senior citizens has come an
increased awareness and openness about many aspects of
aging previously not discussed. Sexuality is one of them.
A survey done in 1996 by Professor Minichiello of the
University of New England revealed that 66 percent of
men and 33 percent of women over sixty-five are sexually
active. The disparity in percentages may not accurately
reflect decreased interest on the part of the women, but
simply the availability of men, since in this age group
women far outnumber men.

The easy availability of information, coupled with the
population bulge of the Baby Boomers, has illuminated
many aspects of life, like menopause, which were previously only whispered about or conducted behind closed
doors. "Sex after 50" is one of these.

In our popular culture, sexuality is associated with
perfect young bodies, preferably trendily dressed and
hyperkinetic in aerobics or sports or some upwardly
mobile occupation. It is not associated with wrinkles,
gray hair, or gravity-pulled guts. But whatever happens
to the wrappings, people retain all their human
emotions, longings, and needs for intimacy at all ages.
Aging without intimacy is a very lonely business. Many
younger people are a little repulsed at the idea of Mom
and Dad having sex, but should instead be more
mindful that they, too, will one day be this age and will
not want to be tucked up on a shelf only to appear for
the grandchildren and otherwise be content to just
quietly wait to die.

It is normal to be interested in sex at any age. And satisfying sexual relationships are defined by the partners in these relationships: they may involve a lot of sensual intimacy, without orgasm, or they may involve very vigorous sexual intercourse. The key is the satisfaction of the partners.

Good health, of course, contributes to good sex, but there are few disabilities that absolutely preclude sex. Heart disease, high blood pressure, arthritis, visual and hearing impairments, even memory loss do not keep you from enjoying a sexual relationship. If you have had a recent heart attack or take cardiac medications, you should ask your doctor how vigorous you can be, and how soon after your attack this can happen. Many cardiac rehabilitation programs now address this issue. If arthritis is a problem, perhaps time your medications in such a way that you can enjoy sex when your pain relief is at its best level. Also remember that sexual excitement and orgasm unleash powerful feelings of well-being and these may actually help to diminish your pain.

Some of the common medications for high blood pressure, heart disease, and diabetes, as well as other conditions, may interfere with the ability to get a good hard-on. If you are taking medicines for any reason and are having difficulties in that department, talk with your doctor—perhaps your prescription can be changed.

Of relevance here too is the common condition of benign enlargement of the prostate gland, that little nut of an organ that embraces the urethra, seminal vesicles, and each end of the vas as it passes into the penis.

Common symptoms of enlargement of the prostate are getting up at night to pee, particularly annoying if this happens several times each night, having to wait for the stream to start, and dribbling, due to only a small amount of urine being able to flow through the narrowed opening. Sometimes there may be blood in the urine (hematuria) and urinary tract infections can occur (see Chapter 17). Acute retention of urine—when the urethra is blocked off altogether—is a painful emergency requiring an immediate visit to hospital and the passage of a catheter. As we'll explain in Chapter 20, benign enlargement of the prostate is most usually treated by a procedure done through the urethra—a TUR, trans-urethral resection—which removes some of the offending tissue. Under a general anesthetic, we add hastily. Further details of this procedure are beyond the brief of our book—we give you some further resources in our appendices.

It is normal as you grow older for your bag of tricks not to be as eager and ready as ever, even if your mind is. It may take longer to get it up; it may be softer and wilt more quickly; orgasm may be shorter and less intense; and a man may be less aware of when he is about to come. However, none of these factors need get in the way if you are open and inventive. Shocking as it may seem to some, orgasm doesn't have to be the aim of a sexual encounter and, more commonly than you might think, only one of the partners may reach climax. What matters is that the couple agree on what is good for *them*.

And speaking of couples, not all elders are in couples. Holy Moly, there is in fact a sexual revolution taking place among the elderly! With the advent of Viagra for men and hormone replacement for women, and the advertisements that celebrate this, older people are now exploring casual as well as committed relationships.

Edith, a sixty-six-year-old widow, was very excited about the idea of "dating" and wanted to get some vaginal lubricant and maybe a little testosterone or tibolone to help her enjoy it even more. She said: "I don't care what anybody thinks. I want some fun and I don't want to cook somebody's meals or wash his socks or clean his bathroom. I'm enjoying my freedom. I got married when I was eighteen and never had a chance to experiment." In fact, a concern of the sexual health clinics is the rise of STDs in the elderly and the lack of education about safe sex in this age group. There's a story—possibly an urban myth—about an eighty-year-old widower, living in a retirement facility in Florida, who discovered Viagra and prostitutes in the same year. He was already a popular guy in the housing complex and now there are ten old ladies with HIV. We don't know if it's true, but it illustrates the problem. Condoms used to be just to prevent pregnancy—at least in some people's minds—and the sophistication of safe, or safer, sex hasn't caught on as quickly as the sex itself.

Mae is eighty-two years old and looks about seventy. Ralph is seventy-two. They've been seeing each other for two years. Recently, Ralph had a heart attack and came to stay in Mae's apartment to recover. Now that he's better, they've resumed their separate living arrangements, but are insepa-rable. Mae says she'd forgotten what it was like to have a man but says: "It's really nice. He treats me like a queen. We still have all of the equipment and just because it doesn't work quite as well as it used to doesn't mean we don't enjoy it." Mae compares herself to a chilli pepper: "Maybe a bit wrinkled on the outside but still red-hot on the inside!"

Remember Evie and Fred from Chapter I? One of

Fred's problems turned out to be his doctor's recent well-meant prescription of antidepressants to help Fred cope with his divorce. There may be an element of depression associated with the many losses one experiences with aging and it may be appropriate to treat the depression ... but that assumption should not be made automatically. One side-effect of antidepressants can be difficulties with erection ... we saw what the treatment did to Fred, combined with a little too much booze. (More about Evie and Fred, and a happy ending, later on.)

Many elderly couples choose to live separately because our social systems penalize them for marrying by taking away the government pension of one (usually the woman). For some, this makes marriage an economic impossibility; for others, it is an insult to lose the money for which you worked for so many years. Some are pressured not to marry by adult children who fear a loss of inheritance if their parent remarries; others are pressured by adult children not to marry because "living together at your age—it's disgusting!" Which, of course, it is not.

> Val and Duncan are a fairly remarkable couple. As Val said to Michele: "We're well paired. My left side doesn't work because I had polio as a kid, and he's blind on the right and has one bad ear. He doesn't walk very well either because of a car accident when we were in our forties. But our other equipment works pretty well and we solve all our problems in bed. We've done this for fifty years and I can't imagine stopping now. Of course, since his heart attack I try to do more of the work. Like lots of folks our age, we've just adapted our habits to fit our conditions."

Hiro and Leslie retired from high-powered publishing jobs five years ago. They are very much enjoying gardening, traveling, and reading together. They visit their children frequently, but also take at least one "exotic" trip each year. Recently they returned from Argentina, where they visited a cattle ranch, among other things. Hiro told Caroline very frankly that he and Leslie haven't had intercourse for probably fifteen years: "I've always been one who thought more about it than I needed to actually *do* it, and when Leslie had her menopause, her interest went way down. Gradually, we've snuggled more and copulated less. Now it doesn't much cross my mind unless I'm watching a sexy movie."

As you can see, the need for intimacy is normal and there is a broad range of ways in which people satisfy this need.

CONDOMS: GETTING IT ON 12

Virginia is recently divorced. She married Ken straight out of high school and has no sexual experience other than in her marriage. Now she suddenly finds herself in the twenty-first century world of dating and sexuality and feels very much like an alien in a strange new world. At fifty-five years of age, the only contraceptive she ever used was the Pill and she has never even seen a condom. And these diseases people talk about! Almost enough to put a girl totally off sex . . . but not quite.

Inge is in first year at college and just met "an incredibly cool guy—he's so sweet." Last night, Inge phoned her Mom and told her about this guy and asked her how to protect herself if she decided to have sex with him. Mom was a little nonplussed, but happy that Inge feels able to come to her with even these very personal questions. Mom told her: "Inge, the first thing to remember is what the ads all say— 'if it's not on, it's not on!'"

Theo's an "incredibly cool guy" in third year at Inge's university.

in order to catch the ejaculated sperm. It is typically made of latex (rubber), although a polyurethane version has recently become available for those people (male *and* female) who have a latex allergy.

The condom is classified as a barrier contraceptive—that is, it forms a barrier between the spurting penis and the cervix of the woman, thereby preventing the passage of sperm into the vagina and cervical canal. It is a reasonably effective method of birth control, 97 percent effective at preventing pregnancy when it is consistently and correctly used. However, the overall pregnancy rate using condoms is something like 15–18 percent. This reflects incorrect and inconsistent use.

An even more compelling reason for using a condom in today's sexual scene is that it is about the only thing we have that allows us to have sex but protects us to some extent from sexually transmitted diseases (STDs). In the 1960s, liberation from the fear of pregnancy by the Pill was celebrated by a couple of generations of free love—free of fear and responsibility. That was all changed as HIV and other nasties hit the scene in the 1980s.

Irene is a young high school teacher. She had lived with the same partner throughout her college years, but broke up just after her final exams when he took up with someone else. To help mend her broken heart, Irene went on a beach holiday with some girl-friends. One night in a bar, Irene met Danny and three double vodkas later found herself in bed with him in his hotel room. She was still taking the Pill following her breakup with Brad so she wasn't going to get pregnant, but oops! she hadn't thought to get herself any condoms. After all, it wasn't as if she had been *planning* to have sex . . . And when Danny didn't produce condoms she was just too embarrassed, and too drunk, and everything was happening too fast to mention them herself. Anyway, she told herself next morning when her friends were laughing about it with her, she surely wouldn't catch anything just from a one-night stand. Wrong! Back home, Irene tested positive for chlamydia, and needed two weeks of antibiotic treatment, just at the time she was starting her first job, before the infection cleared. Fortunately her other STD tests were all negative.

All condoms sold in the United States, Australia, Britain, and most Western countries are required to meet stringent manufacturing specifications, including being subjected to electronic testing to check for holes or other defects. A "water test" is also performed on a random selection from each manufacturing batch—in the United States this means that the condom must withstand one and a quarter cups of water and not leak (the amount in Britain is twelve and a half cups—we're not sure what this implies about English men). An "air burst" test is also done to make sure that a condom can't be blown open. This testing is overseen by the relevant drug and therapeutic goods authorities, including periodic inspections of condom factories and testing of random samples in their own labs (*no*, is the answer to what you're asking, the tests are done by machines, not men). Any sex product that could be construed to be a condom has to meet these requirements.

All condoms are not equal. So-called natural condoms,

made of lambskin or membranes, can protect against pregnancy but may not protect against HIV or other diseases
because the naturally occurring pores in these allow some
microbes to pass through. Some condoms are treated with
the spermicide nonoxynol-9, and this does increase the contraceptive efficiency, as well as possibly adding further
disease protection. We cannot at this time say that it
increases the protection against HIV.

Fancy condoms—ribbed, flavored, colored—are just
cosmetic differences and make no difference to the basic
function. If a guy can put it on his erect penis, then it has
to meet the standards of the country it's produced in.

The term "correctly and consistently" keeps cropping
up. What do we mean? Some couples play Vatican roulette
with the "safe time of the month" and don't use a condom
with every act of intercourse. Some guys whine and plead
that they can't really feel it when they wear a rubber. Poor
babes—then why do they want it so badly? "Consistently" means with *every* act of intercourse. As we saw with
Irene's story, it only takes one unprotected act to become
pregnant or to contract chlamydia, gonorrhea, or HIV. Or
all of the above.

"Correctly" means that the condom fits snugly on the
shaft of the erect penis and that a little air space is left at
the end for the sperm to pool in. More "tips" can be found
at the end of this chapter. The sad fact is that studies show
that only about 17 percent of heterosexuals with more than
one partner use a condom with every act. This is like driving
on black ice without a seat belt. More failures result from
human failure than from condom failure. But let us
acknowledge that, like any safety measure, condoms are
not 100 percent foolproof and sometimes there is a break

or a leak. If this happens to you, don't panic—but consider following our recommendations for emergency contraception (at the end of this chapter) and having STD screening tests (see Chapter 17).

HYSTERICAL TIDBITS

Condom use is centuries old. In records from many ancient and traditional cultures, use of adornments on the penis is mentioned—not for their contraceptive or disease preventive properties, but instead as ways of paying homage to the erect member. An example is the penis sheaths fashioned from gourds by natives of New Guinea.

The earliest true condoms were made of fabric impregnated with whatever substance was thought to prevent pregnancy. Vinegar was once used. These were tied closed at the end. They didn't fit well and were not particularly popular.

Later, progress led to the use of fish skin or animal gut, again tied off at the end. Casanova was rumored to have used a blue silk ribbon on the end of his! Since the knowledge of those days didn't include much about infectious agents, these condoms were reused—often, if one believes the tales of the owner's virility.

The condom is said to be named for Colonel Condom, an army physician attendant upon King Charles II. Allegedly, Colonel Condom made devices from lambs' guts to assist his king, who had an ever-wandering eye for the ladies. As Charles had at least fourteen children by various mistresses, there were clearly defects in the Colonel's design (one wit wrote that "a king should be a father to his people and Charles was certainly father to a good many of them"). The British deny the very existence of Colonel Condom and refer to condoms as "French letters," implying that all such things must be French.

A nineteenth-century New York sausage maker, Julius Schmid, realized the usefulness of his surplus sausage skins, sewn over at one end, for protecting the old sausage. Julius founded a condom company that thrives to this day!

Also in the nineteenth century, developments in rubber manufacturing allowed condoms to be mass produced and become popular. This popularity was enhanced by the development of a liquid latex process in the 1930s and subsequent automation made them very affordable.

CONDOM TIPS

Read these in conjunction with Figure 11.1.

1. Put the condom on correctly. This means placing the condom on the head of the penis and then unrolling it up the erect shaft all the way to the base of the penis. Leave a little air space at the end to collect semen. Make sure that the fit is snug and free of air spaces by smoothing it over the penis toward the base.

2. Never use an oil- or petroleum-based product (e.g. Vaseline) for lubrication. These allow the rubber to weaken and possibly break or leak. If you need a lubricant, use a water-based one, like KY jelly or other products advertised as personal lubricants. Polyurethane condoms are not adversely affected by oils.

3. Be careful not to tear the condom with your fingernails, teeth, or any other sharp object. Be especially careful if the condom is being put on with the partner's mouth that teeth do not tear holes in the condom. (Be aware, too, that most sexually transmitted diseases can

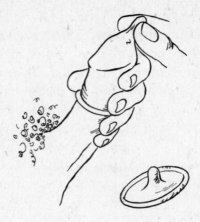

Figure 11.1: Putting on a condom

be passed from Dick to the mouth or throat of a partner performing fellatio, or oral sex. Condoms will provide some protection—see Chapter 17 on infections.) Keep the penis away from the partner's genital area and mouth before putting on the condom because sometimes some ejaculate can leak out before orgasm.

4. After ejaculation, carefully remove the condom by holding firmly to the rolled rim of it and draw it carefully off the still erect penis after withdrawal from the vagina. If you wait until the penis flops, the danger of leaking semen is strong, especially if the condom falls off while still in the vagina. Be sure to dispose of the condom in such a way that no one will be exposed to the semen. A good idea is to seal it in a Ziplock™ bag and place it in the garbage can.

5. Never reuse a condom. You might as well not use one at all. If you are with a new or not well-known partner, watch to see him take the condom from its unbroken wrapper.
6. Don't use a condom if the package seems damaged or if the rubber feels brittle, sticky, is discolored, or is in any other way suspicious. Also, don't use it if it is past its expiration date. Rubber deteriorates and you need to play it safe.
7. Take care of your condoms. Keep them stored in a cool, dry place. Heat or sunlight can damage them. Many women favor the zip compartments in purses and men tend to keep one in their wallets. Don't keep them together with your nail clippers!
8. If you are embarrassed by going into the drugstore to buy condoms, you can also buy them online or by mail. It is easy to find sources online. Be aware that if you are using a library computer for Internet access, they may have a family filter that will block you accessing these sites. If so, ask a friend. Some resources are also provided at the end of this book.

Initially, Virginia was very embarrassed about buying condoms. She went to a pharmacy in a distant suburb. At the checkout, she handed over her basket with aspirin, cold cream, and the red packet of three condoms, fully expecting the salesgirl to wink or smirk or tell her she was too old for that sort of thing. To her great relief, none of that happened—she was just given her change and that was that. People buy condoms everywhere every day, Virginia found.

Inge discovered that she could get condoms from slot machines in the ladies' rooms at the university and in the Students' Union, and that all her friends did this too. She also found that her new love, Theo, was well provided with condoms and completely understanding about her need for protection. The day after he first met Inge, Theo went online on his brother's computer and ordered twelve dozen condoms—he found that they are cheaper in bulk and he was planning to use lots . . . (Incidentally, Inge also followed another piece of her Mom's advice and started on the Pill as well, for contraceptive certainty.)

Even if you are very sure you won't be having sex it's still a good idea to have a condom *just in case*, as Irene's story shows. This especially applies to women, since it is women who experience unwanted pregnancy and women who generally suffer more severe consequences from sexually transmitted diseases. But men too need protection from STDs and the risk of unplanned pregnancy, and should be concerned about their partners' well-being (OK guys, we hear you, we know you mostly are). Having condoms ready for when you might need them is just good sense.

In theory, *both* partners should always take responsibility for the use of condoms in any sexual situation, apart from committed and certain monogamy where some other form of contraception is in use, or pregnancy is wanted, and both partners are free of STDs. In practice, we know it doesn't always work like that. It can be difficult for a young woman, or even an older one, to introduce the topic, and even more difficult to insist on condoms with a guy who doesn't want to use them, especially if she likes him, doesn't want to lose him, and is at the beginning of a relationship. It's best to introduce the subject *very early* before things get too hot and out of control. If you find it too difficult to talk about, then *just produce the condom*—that should make it clear: no glove, no love! And remember, if a guy doesn't care enough about his partner to be concerned about her protection, maybe she should question whether he's really worth it at all.

If you have never put on a condom, regardless of whether you're male or female, it's a good idea to practice first—well before the occasion (um) arises. If you're male, this practice obviously can be on your own erect penis in the course of masturbation. If you're not a penis owner, try a banana, zucchini, or vegetable of your choice, following our directions above. Some enlightened schools teach this skill in Personal Development classes, where certain students have proved better at it than others (hmm). But if you didn't take this class at your school you can always practice at home. If you know how to do it, you will feel more in control when the time does come. Women in the twenty-first century should not feel that knowing how to use condoms, and always carrying them, makes them "cheaper" or "easier," or that it is evidence that they are "asking for it." It's just good sense to be well prepared. And men who always have them available should be regarded by the women who have sex with them as sensible, caring guys.

There is also available a "female" condom, a soft and thin polyurethane sheath that fits inside the vagina and is held by a springy ring visible at the vaginal opening. This provides reasonable protection against both pregnancy and most sexually transmitted diseases. It has the advantage of being able to be inserted well before any sexual activity commences and left in place for some hours afterwards. Its main disadvantage is a tendency to rustle during sex, which can be disconcerting for both partners, and we have to say it has not been very popular so far.

EMERGENCY OR "MORNING-AFTER" CONTRACEPTION

We've put this here to help on occasions of condom failure (and it's always easy to blame the poor old condom), but it applies equally to any kind of contraceptive failure or just to unprotected intercourse at any time. However, it comes with our very strong recommendation that you follow it with some kind of continuing reliable contraception, and that does not include thinking "well, that won't happen again."

The ready-packaged "progestogen-only" morning-after pill levonorgestrel is now available in many countries. This has fewer side-effects (nausea and vomiting) than earlier morning-after pills. If taken within twenty-four hours of unprotected sex, it is 85 percent effective at preventing an unwanted pregnancy. It probably acts by preventing fertilization, but its mechanism is not known for sure. It can be taken up to seventy-two hours after unprotected sex and still be effective, but its effectiveness declines with every passing hour. If vomiting does occur, another dose should be taken as soon as possible.

The only other side-effect is possible light vaginal bleeding before the next period is due.

The older form of emergency contraception consisted of two doses of the pill, with the doses taken twelve hours apart. This often caused vomiting, so some kind of anti-vomiting medication was also given (e.g. Stemetil). Again, it works best when given as soon as possible after unprotected sex.

13 PROBLEMS: MAYBE IT'S FALLING OFF, AND OTHER SCARY SYMPTOMS

The penis and scrotum are covered with skin exactly like the skin elsewhere on the body, so the same skin conditions can occur, and are generally no reason for losing sleep.

Aaron was behaving very strangely. His mother was worried because he was spending an hour at a time in the bathroom and seemed in general to be depressed. In fact, she hadn't had to replace the supply of ice cream once in the past week. Finally she had his dad corner him for a man-to-man talk. "Dad, it's got bumps—they're red and they itch and they're all over my balls," an anguished Aaron told his father. A prompt trip to the doctor led to reassurance. The red bumps were *angiokeratomata of Fordyce*, a big name for small red bumps that may be sore, itch, and bleed. These are not a problem, although they can frighten the uninitiated.

Lexy, a dark-skinned rock musician, turned up one day in the consulting room of one of our colleagues, highly agitated because he'd suddenly found his foreskin had turned white! He was reassured by the doc that this was simply *vitiligo*, a benign skin condition that involves the loss of pigmentation in patches of skin anywhere on the body. It occurs in all ethnic groups.

Craig, whom we mentioned in our first chapter, had a condition called *pearly penile papules*, which can easily be mistaken for genital warts. These are tiny pearly structures, each no bigger than a pin's head, along the ridge (the coronal ridge) just below the glans. They are neatly arranged and, unlike warts, are permanently present. They are perfectly harmless variations on normal anatomy.

Fred, who's now in his fifties, has had a problem all his life with *psoriasis*, especially when he was younger. The patch on the shaft of his penis would come and go—mostly with stress, he thought. Vitamin E cream helped. Any form of skin rash that you can have elsewhere, you can have on your penis or balls. This means eczema, psoriasis, drug reactions, contact dermatitis, and a myriad of others.

Poor Ben suffered terribly in the early months of his marriage. He had a very itchy rash on his penis and balls and even around his anus. He thought it had something to do with marriage until the day the shop was out of the bath soap that the new couple had been using. After a few days with the new soap, Ben was itch-free.

Small cysts can also appear, just as they can anywhere else. *Sebaceous cysts*, which are small smooth flat plaques containing sebum, a creamy yellow fluid, often occur—especially on the scrotum. Only if they are very numerous or become infected do they need removing.

Any *moles* or *freckles* that have been present and unchanging for a long time are benign, but keep an eye on them for any change of color or increase in size, as is recommended for the rest of your skin. Report any such changes to your doctor, and certainly get all newly appearing lesions checked out, as well as anything that hurts, bleeds, oozes, or itches—there are some changes that are precancerous and can occur in the skin of the penis.

Especially in warm climates, in the folds of the skin such as the groin, a bacterium called *Corynebacterium minutissimum* thrives and causes a velvety brown appearance to the skin. This may cause itching and can be treated with antibiotics.

A common cause for silent worry can be a hard translucent swelling on the shaft of the penis. On questioning, this will be found to have appeared after intercourse or masturbation and is a ballooning of the lymphatic channels that have become blocked by this minor trauma. This will go away with no need for help from anyone.

Another common scourge is a *yeast infection* ("thrush", see also Chapter 17), especially on the glans and under the foreskin in uncircumcised men. This is more common in diabetics, men whose partners have untreated yeast infections, uncircumcised men, and those living in warm climates. Washing with mild soap and water, drying well, and using an antifungal cream available over the counter from your local pharmacist should do the trick.

The bottom line with all these symptoms is not to worry—go and see your doctor for a definitive diagnosis and treatment, if warranted, but don't have any nightmares. Dick is not falling off.

The balls also are not immune to various infections. The epididymis, that long coiled tube that leads from the testis into the urethra, is more commonly infected than the testis itself (inflammation of the testis is called orchitis—those orchids again). *Epididymitis* produces, as you might imagine, pain and tenderness and swelling in the affected part, and often fever and a general feeling of being unwell. A urine sample should be taken to identify the bug responsible before starting antibiotics. (Your doctor will want to have a good look first to confirm the diagnosis, and make sure that what you have got is not a torsion, or twisting, of the testis—see the next chapter.) Resting up, firm support of the scrotum, avoiding sex, and pain relief are all clearly a good idea, as well a course of antibiotics.

Orchitis can be an extension of epididymitis, or may be due to mumps or infection in the prostate gland. The treatment is similar to that for infection in the epididymis.

14 KINKY THINGS: HYPOSPADIAS, HYDROCELES, AND OTHER CURLY ONES

Roger was changing the diaper of his week-old son when Wow! What was going on? the baby had a tiny erection and the little hole wasn't winking at him—where was it? Roger knew the child was able to wee, or he wouldn't need a change . . . but this apparatus didn't look at all like his other son's.

He quickly took the baby down to the family doctor, where he was told: "Yes, young Mitchell has *hypospadias*. This is relatively common and is an accident of development. It occurs in about one in every 350 births. You will notice as Mitchell gets a little bigger, that when he has an erection, his little worm will probably have a slight downward curve. This is called *chordee* and almost always goes with hypospadias. It is caused by a fibrous band of tissue that pulls the penis into a curved shape. I'm going to refer him to the pediatric urologist, and when he's a little older—say about a year—he'll be scheduled for a surgical repair. You can see the opening to his urethra just on the underside of his glans, so it is possible that the urologist will be able to repair it in one operation . . . but we'll leave that to him; he's the expert!"

Hypospadias is relatively common and is usually detected on routine well-baby examinations. The skin closing over the passage that forms the urethra is deficient in part and is just replaced by a groove along the underside of the penis. It is usual to try to repair it early in life, before the child enters school, so he doesn't suffer from the remarks of other children.

Hypospadias is usually mild, and men who have undetected hypospadias are able to have intercourse normally and father children. (One well-known historical figure who had hypospadias was the French King Henri II, husband of Catherine de Medici. Henri fathered at least thirteen children, both legitimately and illegitimately.) Obviously, if chordee is severe, intercourse would be impossible; fortunately, this situation is almost always repaired in childhood. Corrective surgery usually results in a penis that looks normal and functions normally. Many women never know that their partner had this condition as a child or had surgery for it.

Why does this happen? There are lots of theories, but no one really knows. Links have been made between things as diverse as vegetarianism in the mother, estrogens in the environment and parental age. But if your child has hypospadias, it is not your fault! We don't know what causes it, therefore, we don't know how to prevent it.

One thing worth noting is that the repair for hypospadias requires as much loose skin as possible, to reconstruct the urethra all the way to the usual place of opening on the tip of the penis. So obviously a little boy with hypospadias should not be circumcised—he needs every bit of skin he can get.

Sometimes, a baby is born with the urethral opening at the junction of the penis and the scrotum. He must be carefully checked for the presence of his testes and, if both are not down in the sac, evaluated for possible ambiguous sexual determination. You may have heard stories in the media of people assigned a sex when young and later being unhappy with their gender. For this reason, gender assessment and assignment are now handled with great care, assessing the chromosomal sex of the child as well as the "eyeball assessment."

What happens if the baby's testes are not down in the sac? First we need to explain that the testes initially begin development up in the abdominal cavity and track down through the inguinal canal in the groin into the scrotal sac. This is completed in most babies by the time of birth, although it may occasionally be delayed up to three months after birth, especially in premature babies. You'll notice that many baby boys have little balls on elastic strings—that is, you can actually see their balls spring up into their groin with the shock of cold air or a startle. This is quite normal because their balls do mostly stay down in the scrotum.

But when the testes are not in the scrotum at all, it may mean that they have never formed—in which case the sex of the baby may need to be determined by testing the chromosomes—or that one or both got lost in the developmental migration from the abdominal cavity down through the groin and into the scrotal sac. This condition is called *cryptorchidism* (hidden orchids!) and it is necessary for the concealed testis or testes to be surgically removed

or brought down into the scrotum because there is a
much-increased risk of testicular cancer later in life if they
are left lurking elsewhere.

There are other forms of congenital (at birth) deformities of the penis, but they are very unusual. They include
the rare incidence of a double penis.

Kimberly recently got the scare of her life: she was
potty training Jamie and he was straining hard. As he
turned a bit red in the face, she saw his little scrotum
blow up like a balloon. It seemed to be only on one
side. Immediately, she snatched him up and called
the doctor. Dr. Hatch came to the phone and very
calmly reassured Kimberly that it was probably "just
a hydrocele" and to bring Jamie in. Sure enough, Dr.
Hatch held a penlight against the skin of Jamie's
scrotum and it looked like a glowing ball. Dr Hatch
said this pretty much confirmed it was a hydrocele.
However, the next step was an ultrasound of the
scrotum.

A hydrocele is a fluid collection within the scrotum. It
should still be possible to feel the testis within the sac,
it commonly occurs on one side only, and it in fact has no
pathological significance. It is present in about 6 percent
of male babies and can occur in adults as well. In the
babies, it is usually the result of a persistent opening of the
tube through which the spermatic cord leaves the abdomen
and goes into the scrotum (see Figure 2.2). This tube,
present in the developing foetus, is called the *processus
vaginalis*. It usually closes off in early infancy. This type of
hydrocele is called a communicating hydrocele. Later in

life, hydroceles may arise from increased fluid production in the scrotum or impaired absorption of this fluid. This is usually a response to some trigger of inflammation in the scrotum, such as a viral illness or an injury.

A hydrocele is not, in and of itself, a cause for alarm. Those occurring later in life will be investigated to be sure that there is no associated pathology, such as a testicular tumor, but usually they resolve themselves with a wait-and-see approach. Many pediatric surgeons repair persistent communicating hydroceles in children; this is a delicate procedure, but is very safe. It is also safe to leave it alone as long as one is sure that it truly is a hydrocele, as a hydrocele has no adverse effect on health or sexual function.

All doctors are aware that a hydrocele can conceal the surgical emergency of a testicular torsion. In this, the testis is twisted upon itself, like a melon on a stalk. This threatens the blood supply to the testis and requires urgent surgical intervention. In this case, the man or boy has excruciating pain in the scrotum and it should be the first thing the doctor thinks of. Fortunately, torsion does not happen often.

Adults can be pretty kinky, too. There is a condition called *Peyronie's Disease*, which occurs in between 0.3 and 4 percent of white men, most commonly between the ages of forty and sixty, although it can be seen as young as thirty and as old as eighty. It is uncommon in African men and virtually unheard of in Asian men.

Gerald was in bed with Deirdre, getting all hot and bothered, when he noticed that his best man *hurt* as it got hard. This was a new one. Good job he could ignore it. When he got up later to pee, he checked himself out and found a very small firm lump in the shaft of his pride and joy. He figured it was probably just an ingrown hair and would go away. But over the next couple of months, the nodule in his penis seemed to thicken more and he continued to have some minor pain whenever he had an erection. He might still have ignored it but one night Deirdre said: "Good god, Gerald, your dick looks like a ram's horn!" (Deirdre was never a very tactful person.) And, indeed, his penis was curved downward ... until her remark deflated him and it curled into a shy little snail.

Gerald's doctor explained to him that, while we don't really know what causes Peyronie's, there seems to be an association with trauma and that it has been historically associated with "excessive sexual inter-course"—whatever that is. In most cases, there is a slow progression of plaque or nodule formation in the shaft of the penis, leading to varying degrees of curvature. Less often, the curvature happens sud-denly and then remains static. There is a spectrum of severity that goes all the way from having painless but palpable plaques in the shaft of the penis to having a curvature so severe that it is impossible for the man to have intercourse.

Gerald was a forty-year-old white man and this was quite typical for Peyronie's. He didn't have any of the other associated risks: he was not diabetic, did not have high blood pressure, and had no problems with soft erections. Peyronie's is a risk for elderly men with soft erections who engage in frequent vigorous intercourse. In black men, it is associated strongly with diabetes. It also may be seen in men who have *Dupuytren's contracture*—a similar fibrous thickening in the palm of the hand, that draws one or more fingers into the palm. None of this was terribly interesting to Gerald; he just wanted to know what could be done.

Medical treatments for Peyronie's have been discouraging, although our favorite peckerchecker Dr. Cohen advises that there is a place for the use of anti-inflammatory drugs, both to relieve pain and to reduce inflammation. He also reports that Verapamil, a heart and blood pressure drug, has been reported to be helpful in Peyronie's, applied as a cream or gel directly to old Jack. We're not sure why this works or how it was first discovered, but if it works, hey, who cares? An anti-fibrosis drug, aminobenzoate (Potaba) has also been used recently with some success. Some other medical approaches can actually cause harm. Viagra or other erectile aids can trigger more scarring. So can steroid injections into the area, which is why these are absolutely contraindicated. Acupuncture has been tried and, although it doesn't do harm, neither does it seem to help. If the pain or curvature is severe enough to warrant treatment, surgical intervention may be helpful. This is done by a urologist.

It is most important for the man with Peyronie's that he and his partner understand that this is not a cancerous or otherwise medically serious condition and that, in most cases, it is not so severe as to interfere with satisfactory sex. Of course, the partner will also need to be sensitive to her man's feelings about this and not, like Deirdre, make jokes or nasty comments.

Certain infections such as gonorrhoea (Chapter 17),

some injuries, and some kinds of surgery can lead to narrowing of parts of the urethra in young and older men, making peeing difficult. Napoleon Bonaparte apparently had such a stricture; his troops were used to seeing him leaning against a tree on the battlefield, waiting patiently for the stream of urine to start. Such difficulty is also a common symptom of enlargement of the prostate gland, a benign but annoying condition that frequently strikes men after the age of fifty or so. In the case of prostate enlargement, it is usual to offer surgery through the urethra (a trans-urethral resection or TUR of part of the offending gland, done by a urologist). Other causes of urethral narrowing may be treated by dilating the tube with instruments of increasing size (these instruments are called bougies, from the French word for candle). In Victorian times, gentlemen who suffered the effects of urethral strictures carried metal catheters for personal dilatation in their top hats! These days the procedure is restricted to the operating theater. If dilatation is insufficient, more extensive surgery by a urologist is required.

These are the most common kinky problems, although we understand that there are some Australian penis puppeteers who can do very kinky things with their appendages . . . but that's entertainment, not medicine.

15 ERECTILE DYSFUNCTION: HAVING A HARD TIME

Ken married Virginia straight out of high school. In their early years together, Ken simply had no idea that sex could cause any difficulties. When Ken even just thought about Virginia he'd find Dick up and rearing to go, and he didn't mind overhearing Virginia telling her girlfriends that he wore his pants out at the zipper, not the knees. In their twenties, they made love every night; by their forties, it had cooled off a little—it was only three or four times per week.

And then Ken had his fiftieth birthday and everything went downhill. To be precise, he and Virginia went off for a weekend to a resort much talked about by their friends to celebrate his fiftieth, and Dick simply failed to rise to the occasion even once, regardless of Virginia's ministrations. The first night, Ken muttered something about being tired from work and went to sleep. Poor Virginia lay awake most of the night, confused and frustrated. The next day and night were even worse. Ken and Virginia were of a generation that found sex easier to do and to joke about than to discuss seriously, and since

Ken wasn't saying anything about all this, Virginia felt she couldn't broach the subject either.

The situation continued once they were back home, and their whole relationship began to fall apart fast. Thinking that Ken no longer found her attractive, Virginia went and ordered several sheer red and black nighties from Frederick's of Hollywood and started putting on makeup to go to bed. She bought satin bed sheets and flavored body oils and really started vamping him. Ken became more and more distressed as she paid him more attention and Dick didn't cooperate. Virginia began to think that Ken had some action on the side and Ken accused her of being unnaturally sexed. Both partners were embarrassed and hampered by their upbringing in freely discussing the problem. Finally, Ken agreed with Virginia's suggestion that they go to see a therapist.

Ken's problems had become apparent on his fiftieth birthday, which made the therapist they had found think that he was having a crisis over his age. Somehow, none of them made the connection that Ken had started taking medication for his high blood pressure within the month preceding his "little problem." To compound the difficulty, his therapist sent him back to his family doctor, saying that he was suffering from depression, and the doctor put him on an antidepressant. The upshot of it all was that Ken couldn't get it up for anything or anyone. By then he *was* truly depressed and felt that he'd been robbed of his essential being as a man. One thing led to another and, sadly, Ken and Virginia were soon divorced.

Two years after the divorce, Virginia met Paul at the home of mutual friends. OK, OK, they were "fixed up." Dating seemed like some strange jungle to Virginia, after so many years with Ken—especially since sexual mores had become so different from what she had known when she was younger. But Paul seemed like a very nice man and they went out for dinner and to the movies several times before he pressed her to "take our relationship one step further."

Now Paul was also divorced, and though he was really turned on by Virginia, he hadn't had sex with a woman for more than five years. He still had regular erections, though—usually in the shower in the mornings—and he just dealt with these quickly himself. Also, Paul hadn't needed to use a condom since he was nineteen: his ex-wife and earlier girl-friends had all been on the Pill. It just didn't occur to him that all those safe-sex messages he'd seen recently might apply to him.

One night, after a romantic candlelight dinner, Paul and Virginia found themselves together in Virginia's bedroom. He was the first man who'd been there, in the apartment she'd bought after the divorce. She felt quite shy, and still uncertain about what she was doing. It just didn't enter her mind that Paul might feel the same way! Paul had brought a bottle of wine and he played with her, taking a sip of wine and giving it to her in a kiss. His hands roved over her body and she began to realize that all her parts were still working and that Paul's equip-ment seemed ready to go. Her girlfriends had taught her the etiquette of this strange new adventure and she had a packet of condoms ready in her bedside drawer. She brought them out at the critical moment and handed one to Paul.

Well, Paul was mortified—first, he asked himself whether he shouldn't have been the one who brought them along. And if she was so well-provided, maybe she was doing this kind of thing all the time . . . she was probably much more experienced than he was, and was no doubt expecting all kinds of tricks. How had he got himself into this fix?

"Oh, sweetie, we don't need to worry about those things at our age," he said hesitantly.

"Maybe, but it's safe sex and I won't have it any other way, Paul," Virginia said, with more assurance than she felt.

Paul fumbled with the packet. Condoms seemed to have changed a lot—this one was colored pink, for a start; they used to be just plain rubber when he was a kid. He decided to ask Virginia to put it on him—it being much sexier that way. She gently started to roll the condom over the glans of his penis when, to the intense dismay of both of them, the penis began to shrivel and shrink. Exquisitely embarrassed, Virginia stood back and just couldn't take her eyes off what a few minutes ago had been a proudly upright spear and was now a sadly limp dishcloth. Paul looked at her, blushed to the roots of his hair, grabbed his clothes, and ran out of the apartment, leaving Virginia in tears.

No, there was nothing wrong with Virginia. Nor was there really anything wrong with Ken and Paul. Impotence, now cutely called "erectile dysfunction," is not uncommon and probably every man has experienced it at least once, though most would rather die than admit it. If this weren't so, would there be so many ads on TV and the Internet for impotence remedies? In fact, there's been media saturation lately about "erectile dysfunction." The company that makes Viagra estimates that erectile dysfunction affects 39 percent of forty-year-old men and 67 percent of seventy-year-old men at some time or another. And, one way or another, what affects men so profoundly obviously affects women too.

Let's also be clear that different people may mean slightly different things when they talk about having this problem. Ivan, who'd been in a relationship with Harold for more than twenty years, worried when Harold at fifty-five no longer wanted sex every night, and went to being a once-a-week man. Ahmed, who is in his sixties, used to have erections very easily but now they take ten or fifteen minutes of direct stimulation to happen. Mary is distressed because Jimmy gets an erection but it's soft and doesn't last long enough for them to have satisfactory intercourse. David awakens with an erection but it quickly subsides without ejaculation, and he can't get one at any other time, no matter how much Belinda stimulates him. There are many more variations on the theme.

Before talking about causes and remedies, we'd best refresh ourselves about how this cute little worm turns into a rampant sword, ready for action.

Normal erections of the penis are caused by a variety of stimuli, as we described in Chapter 3. These can be tactile, like his stroking your breast; visual, like *Playboy* magazine's centerfold; auditory, like phone sex; or imaginative, like the images formed in an erotic daydream. It doesn't matter what turns you on: the mechanism is always the same. The central computer of the brain, acting via the involuntary nervous system, triggers an alteration of the blood flow to the penis. The Swiss-cheesy tissues in the corpora cavernosa relax and allow blood to fill them and engorge the tissue, making the penis thicken and straighten out and up. As long as the circuit of brain—involuntary nervous system—blood vessels on the penis is not disrupted, the penis remains erect. Obviously, the disruption sought by nature is that of ejaculation, after which the blood drains back out of the penis and it flops.

Many things can cause erectile dysfunction. Among the more common are stress, age, common illnesses like diabetes, hypertension, arteriosclerotic heart disease, high cholesterol, smoking, alcohol, marijuana, fatigue, and prescription medications. Among the prescription medications that most commonly affect performance are diuretics and other heart medicines, antidepressants, tranquilizers (too relaxed to get it up!), high blood pressure medications, cholesterol-lowering drugs, hormones, and cancer treatments. Many others will also cause trouble, so always check with your doctor to see whether your particular medication could be causing or contributing to your problem. Some alternative and complementary medicines and health products can also interfere with and potentiate prescription medications too, so always mention these to your doctor.

Three more stories that typify this problem . . .

Sam and Barbara are both in their early sixties, with three grown children and six grandchildren. They were enjoying the freedom of these "mature years" until, two years ago, Sam discovered that he had diabetes and high blood pressure. Last year he had to have a coronary bypass. Until the decline in Sam's health, he and Barbara had enjoyed sex at least once a week. All Sam had to do was to start thinking about sex with Barbara and there was old Willie, ready and able. Now Sam can't get an erection at all. He feels old, useless, and depressed.

David and Belinda are in their thirties, and have been married for five years. Last year they had their first child, Tahlia. This otherwise joyful event was marred by a difficult pregnancy and birth, requiring many extra doctor's visits, a long hospitalization, and lots of worry. Now they have a stack of bills and are doing a credit card shuffle just to stay afloat. Belinda has stopped work to stay at home while the baby is small, and David is working long hours to try to bring in enough to keep them ahead. Now they are cutting back staff at his job and he lives in fear of the little envelope or summons to his supervisor that will herald a layoff for him. He hasn't shared any of this with Belinda, because he doesn't want her to worry. During the first few months after Tahlia was born, both David and Belinda were just too tired to even think about sex, but now that Belinda feels better, she wonders why David seems so disinterested. She tried a couple of times and couldn't turn him on at all. He just falls asleep in front of the TV every night. Is he having an affair?

Fred has been divorced for three years. His wife left him for another woman. At first, he thought it should be no problem for a reasonably attractive fifty-year-old man, who was financially secure and didn't have any terribly bad habits, to find another partner. But the truth is that Fred hasn't had sex since the year before Pat left him. Recently, Fred met Evie on a vacation. He liked her, she seemed interested in him, so he asked her out several times. Their friendship grew, but the more Fred thought about making sexual advances the more nervous he became. One evening he and Evie went to an early evening concert and then stopped off at Nick's bar. Fred had drinks . . . and drinks . . . and drinks. He took Evie back to her place and, lo and behold, his worst fear was realized. Despite kissing and cuddling with Evie on her couch, and his undoing her lacy black bra, it became clear to Fred that the artillery was just not going to fire. He had to get up and say goodnight to a very surprised Evie and go home by himself. Now Fred is depressed and doesn't dare call Evie again. Alcohol "increases the desire and decreases the performance." It decreases inhibitions and makes it easier to get around to the question of sex, but too much will, as you can see, defeat the purpose.

These are just a few examples. Clearly, difficulty with performance increases with age—as the changes Harold and Ahmed are experiencing show—but it can happen to young men too, especially when there is stress (whatever the cause), or when alcohol or drugs are involved. Stress affects the stimulation cycle right at the central computer—the emotion centers in the brain.

Remember that the nerves, arteries, and veins are all

involved in the successful raising of the flag. The blood supply of the penis and the mechanism that allows blood to pool in the corpora cavernosa can be adversely affected by the same things that affect blood vessels else- where in the body—high cholesterol and "hardening of the arteries," or atherosclerosis, and nicotine (so what do you think the Marlboro man is like in bed?). This was what was happening to Jimmy: even though he wanted to go on having sex with Mary as they'd always done, he just couldn't keep it up. His two-packs-a-day habit was affect- ing the blood vessels supplying his penis as well as those in his legs. Maybe there should be a warning about this on packs of cigarettes—something along the lines of "smoking can damage your sex life."

Damage or disease of the veins of the penis can lead to a too-soft and transient erection. A thrombosis or clot in the venous system of the penis can also lead to a painful inability to "get it down" called priapism. This is not common and is associated with diseases like leukemia and sickle-cell anemia. Although it is certainly "up," it is still an erectile dysfunction and interferes with intercourse.

We mentioned the involuntary nervous system as being a necessary part of the stimulation–erection cycle. Because of this, anything that disrupts the nerve impulses through the spinal cord can adversely affect performance.

Jamal is a good example. Jamal was in charge of distribution for one of a national chain of super- markets until the day he was pinned against a wall by a forklift truck. Although he can now walk again and is able to work at a desk job, he has lost the connections in his spinal cord that allowed him to have an erection as a result of any external stimulation including smooching with his new young wife, Elham. He and Elham accept that this is a permanent loss and that Jamal's previous normal sexual function will not return; they are attending counseling to help them seek new forms of sexual expression. (We'll tell you more about this couple in our chapter on injuries.)

Lester had surgery for his prostate at the age of fifty-eight, and had to have the operation through his belly, instead of the more common approach through the penis. He hasn't had an erection since the surgery. He was told of this possible side-effect, but still feels sad. (For more on prostate surgery and its aftermath, see Chapter 20.)

Diabetes is definitely an enemy of Eros. It can cause damage to the blood vessels, both small and large, and to the nerves, and is therefore a very common cause of erectile dysfunction. This was one of the problems Sam experienced. The current estimate is that up to 10 percent of the adult population of most Western countries is diabetic so it is no wonder that Viagra ads are so all-pervasive. If you are diabetic, the best thing is to keep it under strict control and follow your diet. Above all, DON'T SMOKE! (See our note on diabetes and Dick, on page 113.)

Why do we say don't smoke? Nicotine causes constriction of blood vessels and can cause problems in making these vessels unable to respond to the need for increased blood flow. It does this in many organs of the body, but is especially obvious in the penis. (And, while this is particularly important for men who are diabetic because diabetes also adversely affects blood vessels, it also applies to men with heart disease and high blood pressure—indeed, to all men who want to be and stay healthy, like Jimmy.)

Marijuana can also adversely affect getting and sustaining erections. Prescription drugs act in many different ways (depending on the drug) to impede performance. Rather than attempting a review of all these medications, we suggest that you ask your doctor about your particular situation. It's often possible to make a change to your prescription that will improve the ability to get and sustain erections.

Let's look back at Sam, David, and Fred in the light of what we've just discussed. Sam was having somewhat less frequent erections anyway as he got older—and they took longer to come on and were softer than they used to be. At first this wasn't a problem because the changes were gradual, but then he wasn't feeling well and he felt less and less like having sex. After he recuperated from his surgery and felt more like being sexual, the medications for his high blood pressure, high cholesterol, and diabetes, plus maybe some performance anxiety, made it impossible for him to have an erection. Now he just doesn't want to even mention sex to Barbara for fear of letting her down.

Poor David is feeling overstressed by what's going on at work, on top of all their bills, and he just doesn't want to burden Belinda with any of it, so he also feels very alone. He's also concerned, after Tahlia's difficult birth, that Belinda shouldn't have another pregnancy. Add to that the couple of times they did try and failed, and it's no surprise that nothing moves him below. His morning erections, as we've already mentioned, are a normal phenomenon related to brain changes during sleep, and are evidence that if David's stress is relieved then what Belinda used to refer to as his magic wand will be able to wave again.

And Fred? Fred has been so lonely and depressed that his doctor prescribed an antidepressant for him. It helps a lot and probably helped him to be able to go out and meet Evie, but he didn't know that it could interfere with sexual functioning . . . and then he added all that Dutch courage! No wonder things didn't work.

All of these men have initial solveable problems that are compounded by psychological factors. Stress, worry, overwork: all of these are factors that cause difficulty. Add them to a physical problem and a flop or two and almost any man would have tremendous performance anxiety. In the psyche of a man, almost nothing is worse than not being able to get it up. So what can he do and how can his partner help?

Rule number one for the support person is: don't ever, ever laugh or try to joke about the matter—not even from nervous tension. There is no way he can feel humorous about this. Assure him that it is OK, that things will work out, even if you find it very frustrating—otherwise it compounds the problem. Try to plan your sexual times together so that he'll be rested and relaxed. Set the stage with soothingly erotic things like bathing together or giving each other a massage. Suggest that intimacy doesn't always have to lead to penetrative sex—even though you may hope that eventually this will be possible.

Make sure that, if you use alcohol or recreational drugs together, it is not very much—a little may heighten the libido but too much definitely makes for a limp noodle.

If your house is like Grand Central Station, it may be worthwhile to rent a motel room; consider it reasonably cheap therapy! If you feel that there are medical reasons for his inability to perform, or if you've tried what you can do with no success, get him to a doctor—there's no need for either of you just to accept what can be helped. Check first, though, that the doctor you choose has a thorough knowledge of male sexual functioning and is up to date with all investigations and treatments. Most men will feel more comfortable in this situation with another man, but there are many women doctors who are first-rate practitioners in this field, and some male doctors feel surprisingly uncomfortable discussing sexual matters with patients. We provide a list of suggested addresses at the end of this book.

Investigation should include a thorough medical history and examination for all the possible causes of erectile dysfunction that we've mentioned. It may also include nighttime testing in a sleep lab or with devices provided for use at home, to see whether those nocturnal erections we told you about back in Chapter 3 are occurring. Strain gauges placed around the base and below the glans measure changes in the diameter of Dick while his owner hopefully dreams happily away. In practice now, most doctors are likely to eliminate or treat any disease and then try Viagra—more about Viagra shortly.

On the other hand, it might be that your partner really isn't too bothered by the lack of an erection. Frank discussion about each other's desires is vital here. Many older couples do reach a point in their relationship where they still want to be close, but no longer express that closeness sexually. The world still turns. Alternatively, many women can be completely satisfied by sex that doesn't require the "jade stalk" to be like "a plough in spring," as the pillow books written by the Taoists over the past few centuries so prettily describe it. Oral or hand stimulation of the clitoris by one or both partners can produce orgasm for a woman and this can be rewarding for a man even though he does not climax himself. Vibrators—available in all sizes, shapes, and colors in "adult" shops, by mail, or ordered online—are also useful in this situation. There are no rules here: the important thing is to be as open and honest as possible with each other about your needs and feelings.

Now on to the many devices and concoctions that have been available over the years to help a limp member become—and remain—stiff, if not actually tumescent. Most of these have proved of dubious or minimal effectiveness.

Health food stores sell multiple products that proclaim their ability to increase male potency. They are often called names like "Male Toner" or "Invigorate." Among them are products containing macca and horny goat weed (yes, it really is called that!). These are current favorites and may act as mild aphrodisiacs, stimulating interest but not necessarily ability. Macca is probably safe, but it is more difficult to find reliable information about horny goat weed.

A herbal remedy called yohimbe has been available for as long as we've been in practice. Its origin is Rubaceae and related trees and it is related to the old-time blood pressure medicine Rauwolfia. Yohimbe is listed in some pharmaceutical directories and is described as successfully treating impotence of vascular or diabetic as well as psychogenic origin. In the United States and Britain it is available by prescription. Side-effects can include nausea, dizziness, and nervousness. It acts on the involuntary

nervous control of the blood vessels. Yohimbe is contraindicated in people with kidney disease and should not be
used by those with ulcer disease histories. It also shouldn't
be taken together with psychoactive drugs, like antidepressants. You can talk to your doctor about this.

Advertised in some "home health" catalogues are
adjustable rings—kind of like bracelets—to put around
the base of an erect penis to keep it that way; they are
readily available and quite cheap. Little information is available in the medical literature about them, but one can
immediately see the danger of inadvertently damaging the
veins under the skin by tightening the "bracelet" too
snugly— a little like causing clots in varicose veins by tight
bands around the calves. While they are less likely to cause
any harm in younger men, and may be amusing for themselves and their partners, we wouldn't advise their use for
older men—especially those with diabetes or vascular
disease—because of the possibility of further damage to
the blood vessels. (One suggestion for dealing with the
problem of an erection that starts to sag before intercourse
has reached a satisfactory climax, and which worked for
Mary and Jimmy, is for her to hold the base of his penis
during thrusting—this has the happy double effect of
involving her in stimulating him, while he can direct her if
the pressure is too little or too much. It's worth trying,
anyway.)

Surgeons are eminently practical people, and they have
come up with several devices to implant into the penis to
make it erect. Some of the early attempts quickly flopped
because they gave a man a permanently erect rod, and this
was both an annoyance and an embarrassment. The
latter, more successful ones insert tubes into the corpora

spongiosa and a small saline-filled reservoir into a space behind the abdominal wall. A turn-on mechanism is implanted in one side of the man's scrotum, which he can discreetly trigger so that the saline in the reservoir will squirt into the tubes and make the penis erect. He turns it off the same way, fingering the trigger in his scrotum. A truly bionic man, don't you think? The main problem with most of these is coordinating desire with the erection mechanism. In the "normal" situation, of course, the two just happen together. There is also a small risk of leaking, mechanical failure, and infection.

Another type of vacuum device literally pumps up the penis—it is an apparatus that fits over the penis and pumps with a suction action, with the vacuum produced sucking blood into the penis. A soft rubber ring is placed over the base of the shaft to maintain the erection, and can be left in place for thirty minutes. The vacuum pump has the advantage that invasive surgery is not required, but its effects are generally less successful than prostheses—it works best for men who are able to achieve at least partial erection themselves, as otherwise the portion of the penis between the rubber ring and the body remains floppy even though the main part of the shaft is hard, an effect that can be disconcerting. Clearly, too, a certain amount of preparation time is required, so spontaneity and foreplay may go out the window. But vacuum devices may be suitable for men who need to take nitrates for heart conditions and therefore should stay away from Viagra (see next page).

On to drug therapies. The first drug therapy specifically approved for treatment of impotence was *alprostadil*, known by the trade names *Caverject, Edex,* and *Muse.* Caverject and Edex are injected by the man (or his willing partner) into the corpora cavernosa anywhere from five to twenty minutes before they expect to commence action. The erection will usually last up to one hour, although a possible unfavorable consequence can be a prolonged erection of up to six hours or priapism (an erection lasting longer than six hours). This is not the occasion for joy that might be imagined by the uninitiated. Prolonged erection or priapism can lead to penile fibrosis and permanent impotence or deformities of the penis. Because of these risks, people with conditions that can be associated with priapism, such as sickle-cell anemia or trait, leukemia or multiple myeloma, or deformities such as Peyronie's (see Chapter 14), should not use alprostadil in any of its forms. Muse acts in the same way as Caverject or Edex, but is available as a suppository that the man inserts into his urethra. This drug is excreted through the lungs and its excretion is somewhat affected by lung disease. Obviously, anyone using this not only has to be given a prescription, but also needs to be taught how to administer it.

Now—trumpets and drum rolls—for *Viagra,* or *sildenafil,* the darling of TV and magazine advertising, stockholders, and many men. Pharmaceutical giant Pfizer is also undoubtedly orgasmic about the dollars rolling in. However, whatever one may think of the profit motive that is so obviously behind it, Viagra has been a true advance in treating problems of potency, or erectile dysfunction, converting many a three-and-a-half-inch floppy to a hard drive.

Viagra acts in a complex biochemical way to restore the normal physiological response to sexual stimulation. It increases the level of a chemical called *cyclic guanosine monophosphate* (cGMP), which relaxes the smooth muscle in the walls of the blood vessels in the penis and restores the ability of those blood vessels to fill the spongy cylinders with blood. This is clearly very different from the previously available treatments. With implants or injections, the man was set to go even if he had no compelling interest— a hole in a woodpile would do, as they say. With Viagra, if he "has a headache," his little man will not stand up and beg.

Viagra also has the convenience of being orally administered in an average dose of 50 milligrams and being available in the bloodstream within an hour after swallowing. It remains active for about three to five hours after this. This means that a man can swallow his pill if things are looking promising, enjoy foreplay, and be hot to trot. (With the cost of Viagra, though, sex may not be the final note in a pleasant evening—it may *be* the date.) It is interesting that in many countries the relevant committees were very quick to extend prescription coverage to Viagra, whereas many have held out against the birth control Pill for many years, and others took a long while to approve tibolone, a hormone replacement that improves lost libido in older women.

Many scientific studies have been done evaluating such things as visual sexual stimuli (i.e. the *Playboy* response), and scoring responses by the International Index of Erectile Function. These tests were conducted with several hundred men and did not differentiate between different causes of erectile difficulty. The results have been reported in such distinguished journals as the *Lancet* of London and the *Journal of the American Medical Association.* The outcome is that Viagra is significantly better than a placebo in improving the frequency of vaginal penetration, maintenance of the erection, orgasmic satisfaction, satisfaction from the act of intercourse, and "overall satisfaction," according to the men surveyed. (It's not clear what the partners of these men felt about all this; questionnaires were provided for the partners but only 25 percent filled them out.)

Viagra is *not* an aphrodisiac. That means that if the interest is not there, Viagra will not supply it—it is not a means to restore a flagging relationship. It is also obvious from the studies that, while Viagra will significantly improve the erectile response, it doesn't return it to a man's youthful levels. And it seems that the responses are still lower than "normal," whatever that is. The important thing is that the partners in a relationship be able to express themselves sexually and lovingly. Viagra can help them to do this, but it's not the only factor involved.

Some side-effects have been reported. Headache, facial flushing, indigestion, and some visual disturbance (seeing a bluish tinge around objects) are the most common, but these have been reported by only a small percentage of men. Few men stop taking Viagra because of them.

What about the reports of sudden cardiac death associated with the use of Viagra? These have not been numerous and need to be seen in the context of naturally occurring sudden cardiac death in men over forty during sexual intercourse. This is the origin of so many jokes about "death in the saddle." Obviously, Viagra should be prescribed by a doctor who either knows the health of the particular man very well or who makes it their business to check him out thoroughly before prescribing it. Some men will have health conditions that make it unsafe either to take Viagra or to have sex, or they may be taking medications that are unsafe together with Viagra—notably the nitrates commonly prescribed for heart disease. Some medications may be changed, allowing the use of Viagra; others may not. In men who suffer from kidney or liver disease, extreme care, and possibly lower doses, will be needed.

Generally, 50 milligrams a day is a sufficient dose—some men need 100 milligrams, but more than this should not be taken in any twenty-four-hour period.

As you may be aware, there are many Internet sites offering Viagra. Sure, these have the advantage of keeping the matter relatively private between you and your computer if you decide to purchase Viagra this way. However, a recent survey showed that only about a third of these sites sought any medical history from the men contacting them or had a doctor review that information. Only half provided any medical information about the drug, and less than half explained that taking nitrates is an important contraindication to Viagra. What's more, less than half bothered to ask whether the man concerned actually had erectile dysfunction! As we've explained, Viagra is not an aphrodisiac but fills a specific deficiency in the process of erection. Buying online (or anywhere else) should only take place in conjunction with at least an initial physical check and discussion with a doctor to rule out or treat the health problems we've discussed.

We should also mention here *Cialis* (generic name tadalafil), recently available as a "second-generation" treatment for erectile dysfunction. Cialis works just like Viagra, but according to trials and scientific studies so far available, lasts longer (at doses of up to 25 milligrams) and has less side-effects. Cialis can be effective for up to thirty-six hours, and has been promoted as increasing the opportunities for spontaneous sexual activity. Possibly not everyone would see this as an advantage, but you can take your pick! Side-effects have included headache and indigestion, but not the visual disturbance sometimes reported with Viagra. Side-effects are usually minor and occur in only a small number of men, and to date there have been no reports of serious heart problems with Cialis.

While popping pills may be something a man wants to keep to himself on a first occasion with a new partner or in a casual encounter, in any permanent relationship it is clearly better if the partner concerned is fully aware of what he's taking and how it works, and understands the possible side-effects. Taking Viagra (or Cialis for that matter) may make things less spontaneous than they used to be, but so what? It's just a matter of adjusting and finding new ways of sexual expression together.

At the end of the day, these drugs are currently the safest and most effective treatments available to us for erectile dysfunction. They have advantages of convenience, oral administration and control of erection by normal mechanisms of interest and arousal. Certainly Viagra proved useful for Sam—after Barbara finally marched him back to their family doctor and insisted they talk about it. Willie is now as willing as ever.

We thought we'd mention, too, that Ken and Virginia's son guessed what his dad's difficulty might be and talked with Ken's doctor. At the next visit, the doctor asked Ken about it all, made some changes to his blood pressure pills and prescribed Viagra. Ken worked up his courage and phoned Virginia for a date. It was great, and within six months they had remarried. And Paul? After some hesitation, he also went to see his doctor who prescribed Viagra and had a long chat with him about condoms. The last Virginia heard, Paul was seeing a lot of a very nice woman he works with.

We'll also tell you about David and Belinda. One day recently, David was called to the boss's office . . . to be told that he'd got a promotion and salary rise! He rushed home to Belinda with a bottle of champagne and later that evening . . . bingo!

Finally, you'll be glad to hear that one of Evie's friends got Evie and Fred together again at a wine-and-cheese gathering, only this time without so much *vino*. The outcome is that Fred is off his medication and they've booked a tour together to Hawaii.

DIABETES AND DICK

Diabetes is an extremely common chronic condition and at least 50 percent of diabetic men experience some sexual dysfunction, though many will be reluctant to complain of it, even to their family doctor. However, if diabetes is well managed and sugar levels controlled, the aftereffects including sexual dysfunction can be minimized.

Organic sexual problems may result from diabetes, but note that the sexual problems experienced by men with diabetes are the same as those in the general population, though some conditions are more common amongst diabetics. Equally, sexual problems in diabetic men, like those in non-diabetics, are likely to have a psychogenic as well as an organic component.

It is normal to have some changes in sexual functioning with age, as we describe in Chapter II, and it is important that men with diabetes be aware of these and not attribute everything to their diabetes.

Erectile dysfunction occurs in 40–70 percent of diabetic men—three times the rate in the general population—and starts at a younger age. Fifteen percent of thirty-year-old diabetic men have some degree of erectile difficulty. This is due to nerve damage so that the nervous pathways we've described for erection don't function properly; arteriosclerosis, so less blood flows into the penis; and damage to the veins that hold the trapped blood during an erection so it leaks out. Cigarette smoking, uncontrolled high blood pressure, and high levels of blood fats are also risk factors often present in diabetic men that can increase the incidence of erectile dysfunction.

Some drugs taken by diabetics may also contribute to erectile dysfunction. These include thiazides, beta-blockers, antidepressants, simvastatin, and glucocorticoids.

It is important for diabetics to have appropriate diagnosis and ongoing management of their condition, preferably by a family physician or diabetic team. Good sugar control, lowering of blood fat levels, attention to diet and exercise are all essential. Expert help from a sex counselor and the prescription of Viagra may be needed, but only after attention has been given to all these basic health measures.

Premature ejaculation is a common problem in young men anyway, and it is important that young diabetics don't see it as a complication of their diabetes, as this may make it worse. Delay in ejaculation can also occur as a result of diabetic nerve damage.

Peyronie's Disease is more common in diabetics (see Chapter 14), and infections are also generally more prevalent in diabetics. Attention to hygiene is therefore very important, to reduce the chances of balanitis (bacterial infection beneath the foreskin and on the glans) and yeast infections like thrush. Antibiotic or antifungal treatment may be needed.

PREMATURE EJACULATION: "ROGER AND OUT" 16

Premature ejaculation is a common sexual dysfunction. In fact, probably every man experiences this at least once in his sexual life, though most wouldn't admit it. Definitions of this problem have varied greatly over the years and among the sexperts, with an earlier definition being ejaculation before penetration or within thirty seconds of penetration. Obviously, people asked: "Well, what about thirty-five seconds?" and "How can I tell without a stopwatch?" or quipped "Somehow I forget to time it." Today the definition is ejaculation (and the subsequent return to the flaccid state of the penis) too quickly for the partner to experience pleasure from the episode of intercourse. This is a better definition, but is also not perfect. We suspect that, even without a perfect definition, couples know when they are having a problem in this area. And if they do not know, either because of lack of experience or because their relationship is otherwise so fulfilling in its entirety, then who are we to tell them that they have a problem?

Jim and Marilyn had been married for fifteen years. For the first two years, they experienced wonderful sex and then Marilyn's father died and her mother moved in with them. Sex became a bit more subdued. Three years later, Jim's dad died and his mother also moved in; the mothers were alternately good friends and bitter rivals, and this took up a great deal of Jim and Marilyn's emotional energy. Sex became a quickie when and how they could. It felt almost like being guilty teenagers. Two years ago, the moms announced that they felt just too cramped in this small apartment and were moving together to an independent living facility, and "no, it's no use trying to talk us out of it. We don't want to hurt your feelings, but we've already made all the arrangements."

Jim and Marilyn felt conflicted; they felt a vague sense of having failed in a duty and a huge relief that they could be on their own now. In fact, perhaps it was not too late to have children.

The first weekend on their own, Jim brought home flowers and a special bottle of wine and Marilyn cooked their favorite meal. They took a long leisurely bath together and arrived in bed with a good head of steam going. And then, spurt, flop. Later in the week, a more spontaneous performance ended in the same anticlimax. Instead of building a wall of silence, Jim and Marilyn got up out of bed and cuddled on the couch and discussed what to do about "our problem." Their answer was to buy a vibrator. Any time intercourse was truncated by Jim's coming too soon, he brought Marilyn to orgasm with the vibrator. This worked very well for them and within six months they rarely had to use the vibrator because Jim had become accustomed to again having the luxury of time.

The physiological basis to premature ejaculation is an inability for a man to voluntarily delay his sexual responses. Most men can delay orgasm—"hold back"— for some time while thrusting before ejaculation becomes inevitable. The man who has a problem with premature ejaculation cannot do this. All sorts of psychological theories, Freudian and otherwise, have been proposed to explain this. Indeed, whole books and reputations have risen and fallen on this subject! The most sensible explanation is that the man's previous sexual experiences have been frequently hasty and furtive (remember the backseat of the car at the drive-in?) and may have been associated with guilt or a fear of discovery; his responses have therefore been programmed to fit these circumstances. Most men will have occasional episodes of coming too quickly, usually associated with environmental factors of some sort. Certainly premature ejaculation is often a problem at the beginning of a relationship, associated with the high levels of excitement with a new partner.

Jenny and Don were happily married with two small children who used up much of their energy. They would fall into bed at night, exhausted, with little energy for sex. Even so, they managed to have one or two "quickies" each week—usually in the early morning hours, keeping one ear cocked for sounds from the children's room.

One fine weekend, Don's sister took the kids for Saturday night. Don and Jenny were so looking

forward to this long lazy Sunday morning in bed—
just them and croissant crumbs! And all was perfect,
right up to the denouement, when Don just could
not hold back.

So what is the difference between a quickie and premature ejaculation? Most relationships combine quickies
with more leisurely sex and a quickie is a mutually agreed
need to have sex, but to be quick about it. This can be
because of children or in-laws or schedule demands, or
any of a thousand other reasons, including the fact that
it's fun in itself, but it *is* quick sex with no expectation of
anything else. Premature ejaculation is quick sex because
of an inability to prolong it. In both cases, the woman
can be brought to orgasm by other means if she is not
satisfied.

How can the problem be fixed? Early approaches
centered on a man training himself to think about something else during sex. Can you imagine trying to keep your
mind on football scores or mathematical equations or
listing the presidents of the United States in sequence
while you are in the midst of intercourse? Anyway, that
was the advice. But, just as we might have predicted, it
actually worsened things by making the man nervous and
guilt-ridden by his failure to perform these mental acro-
batics. It was also suggested that he use distractions such
as biting his lip or pinching himself—this was equally
ill-fated.

There are a few products around designed to be
applied to or smeared on the upstanding member in order
to prevent premature ejaculation. The common ingredient
of all of these is a local anesthetic intended to diminish

sensation in the skin. Our colleague Dr. Cohen assures us that he has had success in prescribing this treatment, with the gel being smeared on thinly as soon as Oscar begins to strut his stuff. A word of warning: the emphasis is on *thinly*. Sex under anesthesia? Seems to us it could be a case of throwing the baby out with the bathwater, particularly if some gets smeared on the female partner as well . . .

The only methods that are really helpful enlist both partners to be part of the solution. Masters and Johnson, in their book *The Pleasure Bond*, emphasize the need for intimacy in a sexual relationship—which means time to talk, holding each other, pleasuring each other in ways that are sensual without necessarily being sexual, and not making sexuality a goal-oriented exercise, with mutual penetrative orgasm as the goal. This is not only wise, it is extremely practical advice. More time should be spent in foreplay and mutual exploration. Initially, a pact can be made not to attempt penetration at all, but rather to bring each other to orgasm by manual or oral stimulation or the use of sex toys like vibrators or dildos. If this attempt to alleviate performance anxiety and increase intimacy is not adequate, the couple should seek the help of a credentialed sex therapist.

Such a therapist will start by taking a full history and will want to eliminate any medical problems causing premature ejaculation. If he or she is not a physician, the couple will be referred to their doctor for this purpose. Depression is one condition that can make a man quick to trigger. In this case, the use of antidepressants for a few months may help. (It's also worth noting that some of the more recently introduced antidepressants have proved helpful for men with premature ejaculation, even when depression didn't seem to be a problem. But these should only be used after consultation with your family doctor and/or a sex counselor.)

Next, the program of increasing intimacy and communication that we've mentioned begins. Once the couple are very comfortable with each other's bodies and in communicating with each other about their needs, the therapist will begin teaching them a squeeze technique, illustrated in Figure 15.1. This involves the couple sitting facing each other. The woman stimulates the man's penis with her hand and, as his penis visibly engorges and rises, she squeezes him firmly just below the glans—her thumb on the underside, two fingers on the top—maintaining pressure for about five seconds. This doesn't hurt and the pressure can be quite firm. The urge to ejaculate is lost and then, after a few seconds, the couple repeat the process, continuing several times before ejaculation is permitted. This technique is practiced repeatedly over several weeks before any vaginal penetration is attempted and, initially, vaginal penetration is done without any thrusting. Finally, the couple move on to full intercourse. During all of this, the man may stimulate the woman's clitoris or vagina. This technique "unlearns" premature ejaculation and has a good success rate.

Peggy is a divorced math teacher. Andy is the physical education teacher in her school and he is a real hunk. Peggy's been flirting with Andy for several weeks and he seems to like her, so why hasn't he asked her out? Eventually, she bit the bullet and just asked him along to a football game. How could he say no? They had a few more dates and finally she got him to come in for "coffee" after a night out. Everything was great until they hit the sack—when Andy proved to be a sprinter: quick to the finish line. Peggy was very disappointed, as Andy could see. Fortunately, Peggy was also very sensible and analytic, and she valued this burgeoning relationship, so she suggested they see a sex counsellor. Andy was initially taken aback since this was not yet a long-term, committed liaison, but then he thought: "Hey, what's there to lose?" He'd had this problem ever since his first girlfriend, Madge. Madge was deeply religious and would pray for forgiveness and urge him to hurry every time they had sex. He had really liked Madge, but was driven away by this.

Peggy and Andy went to see a sex therapist who was quite untroubled by the fact that they had just

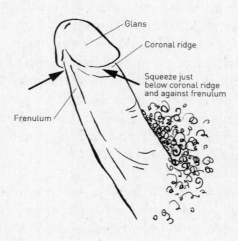

Figure 15.1: Squeeze technique for treatment of premature ejaculation

begun a relationship. They embarked on the course of treatment just described and found greatly increasing satisfaction, not just in the bedroom but in being together in other ways. At the time of writing, they are still together.

COITUS INTERRUPTUS

At this point it seems logical to mention coitus interruptus, coitus obstructus, and coitus reservatus. These are further along the spectrum from trying to overcome premature ejaculation in that, by using these techniques, the object is to control ejaculation for purposes of contraception or, in the case of Tantric Yoga, to achieve a higher state of bliss. Needless to say, they are difficult to practice and we would not advise anyone to rely on these techniques as their sole method of birth control.

Coitus interruptus is the technique in which the man pulls out from the vagina when he feels the inevitability of ejaculation. Now one problem with this, besides the obvious timing problems, is that often a little seminal fluid and sperm leak out before full ejaculation and all it takes to fertilize an egg is one sperm. Also, this usually leaves the woman hanging on a cliff, and both partners feeling less than satisfied by the experience.

Mary was a sweet sixteen-year-old who came to Michele's office for prenatal care—she and her boyfriend Bruce had been using coitus interruptus as their means of contraception. Mary believed Bruce, who was all of seventeen, that "sure, I can control it; no problem."

Coitus obstructus is fully engaging in intercourse while at the same time pinching the shaft of the penis in such a way as to close off the urethra, forcing the ejaculate into the bladder. Frankly, we cannot believe anyone is really able to do this regularly, and we imagine it would be pretty painful!

Coitus reservatus is full intercourse, presumably until the woman comes to orgasm, while holding back from climax—apparently by concentrating the mind on other things. This is practiced in Tantric Yoga, but it takes that type and level of discipline and training. Clearly, this is not for casual sex.

We should also mention another problem that is more common in older men or in men who have had surgery of the prostate or urethra. This is called *retrograde ejaculation* and is characterized by a lack of external ejaculation with part or all of the ejaculate going into the bladder. As one jokester put it: "The charges get reversed." Orgasm is experienced, but with a slightly different feeling owing to the lack of a feeling of fullness in the urethra—Sam, who had prostate surgery in his sixties, described it as "now a one-stage procedure whereas it used to be a two-part performance." One study reports that about 62 percent of men experience this problem after prostate surgery done through the urethra, and it is generally more common in men with diabetes. See more about this in Chapter 18, on infertility.

17 INFECTIONS: BUGS, BUMPS, DRIPS, AND ITCHES

We'll spend most of this chapter talking about sexually transmitted diseases (STDs), since not only is Dick directly involved in transmitting most of these, but the penis is often the first site of infection. Unhappily, despite intense campaigns aimed at safe, or safer sex, millions of people every year contract one or more of these, the vast majority because they have had unprotected sex with more than one partner, or their partner has done so. We can't emphasize too strongly the message of our chapter on condoms—no glove, no love!

But, you say, aren't most of these trivial infections that can be nipped in the bud these days with antibiotics? Isn't it worth taking the risk if it means not having to bother with condoms? Not so. Extensive use of antibiotics has made some bugs—especially strains of the gonococcus that causes gonorrhea—immune to many antibiotics. Herpes and HIV are not, at the time we write, curable by any antibiotic. And, while some bugs causing STDs—such as hep B or Donovanosis—practice "equal opportunity," affecting males and females in similar ways, others like chlamydia engage in "affirmative action" as far as women are concerned, causing severe and silent damage before the woman even knows she's been infected. For this reason, we make no apology for providing a lot of information about how STDs affect women. By far the best protection from all of the diseases we're about to describe, if you're not insterested in abstinence or certain monogamy, is the careful and consistent use of condoms.

At the end of this chapter, we also include some infections that are not sexually transmitted.

GONORRHEA

Gonorrhea is caused by a lover-ly little bug—pairs of little round bacteria known as cocci. It has been around for a very, very long time and remedies are mentioned in Egyptian papyrii dated from 3500 BCE. In the Old Testament (Leviticus 15), rituals of atonement are detailed for "him who has a discharge and for him who has an emission of semen, becoming unclean thereby; also for her who is sick with her impurity; that is, for any one, male or female, who has a discharge, and for the man who lies with a woman who is unclean." These rituals had to do with cleanliness, and avoidance of contaminating others for prescribed periods of time, as well as making sacrificial offerings to God.

Hippocrates, around 400 BCE, recognized that this was an affliction associated with sexual acts, but it was Galen, a Greek physician around 200 CE, who called it gonorrhea, for "flow of seed."

This disease has been called by many names—the clap, drip, Jack, a dose, gleet, morning drop, running range and, most descriptively by the French from the fourteenth century, *chaude pisse*, or hot piss. Hot piss is very much how it feels to the poor man who attempts to empty his bladder through a urethra inflamed with gonorrhea. Characteristically, a man will have symptoms within three to nine days of his exposure to the disease—by having sex with someone who has the clap. Only 10–15 percent of men will *not* have symptoms. An affected man will first experience a burning sensation whenever he tries to take a leak and then notice a creamy drip from his penis. How much drip there is can vary from person to person.

Left untreated, the disease will invade farther up into the urethra and into the neck of the bladder and the prostate. He will feel that he has to pee all the time and urgently—no delay or he may wet himself. As the disease progresses, the urine may be blood-tinged. By contrast, a woman may have few symptoms other than an increase in her vaginal discharge, with or without a little burning, which she may think is a variation on normal. If the illness spreads upward through the uterus into the Fallopian tubes, the woman is usually quite ill with pelvic inflammatory disease (PID) and sterility may result.

Emma was a young mother in her thirties. She used the family planning clinic for her women's health needs and had had a routine STD screen done with her annual Pap smear. To her doctor's consternation, Emma's culture came back positive for gonorrhea. She was notified to come in for treatment and the clinic nurse told her that her husband should also come for testing and treatment. Emma denied any other sexual partners. The day of her appointment came and so did Joseph, Emma's husband. Joseph was more than irate; he was dangerously angry—with the clinic staff! "How dare you say that I gave this to my wife. Your tests must be wrong. Or else she got it from a toilet seat. It couldn't be me, I'm perfectly OK." Now, you know, that old toilet seat possibility just isn't possible—the organism doesn't survive outside a warm human body.

Emma had always struck the nurse as a very meek soul, but the following week she brought a much-chastened Joseph back to the clinic. Seems that Joseph goes out of town every week to sell hairdressing products and a few weeks back he was stuck overnight with a broken-down vehicle and, well . . . his hotrod had been where it shouldn't have gone. As it happened, he had some dental work a few days after he returned from that trip and a dose of penicillin to cover it must have also treated the disease for him—but not before he had infected his wife. It was just lucky for Emma that her checkup was scheduled at this time.

Does gonorrhea go other places in the body? You bet. Keith was a young bartender who came into the emergency room once where Michele was working, complaining of a hugely swollen and hot knee and generally not feeling well. All of the causes of an acute arthritis were thought of and tested for but the payoff was the fluid drawn off Keith's knee. When it was stained in the lab and looked at under the microscope, there were all those cute little red bacteria, two by two, in the white cells. This wasn't too surprising—gonococcal arthritis is the commonest manifestation of gonorrhea outside the sexual organs. Less commonly, and much more seriously, gonococcal meningitis or pericarditis or hepatitis can occur, or a bloodborne septicemia (blood poisoning). These are very serious illnesses, but are fortunately much less common than garden variety gonorrhea.

More common, and often overlooked, are infections in the mouth or anus. These are also nice moist mucous membranes and the little gonococci love warm, moist environments. In fact, they can't live in environments that aren't warm and moist—hence, no toilet seats.

Some rash young men may find that they have a rash, as well as the other symptoms we've mentioned. In fact, Keith had a rash and this helped alert Michele to tap his knee and stain the fluid to look for *Neisseria gonorrhoea*—the proper name for this bacterium.

Since 1937, when sulfonamides were first introduced, we have had effective treatment for gonorrhea. Before that, many things were tried in centuries past and some seemed to have low-level efficacy, while others were harmless at best and dangerous at worst. Washing with gin was one measure thought to prevent infection and may have been mildly effective. In the 1950s, we found that penicillin was incredibly successful in treating gonorrhea, with one test subject being infected and cured three times in one week. (We hope he had the fun as well as the infection.) However, in the 1960s and 1970s, there were world pandemics of gonorrhea and resistance to penicillin and sulfonamides resulted. Penicillin is still the drug of choice for nonresistant gonorrhea, but other antibiotics may need to be used.

It is very important that any discharge from the penis be investigated; this usually involves a swab being taken for staining and culture, but there is also a simple urine test available now. In most Western countries, gonorrhea is a reportable illness by law, so any positive test results are automatically sent to your local Department of Health. A public health worker will contact you to find out who may have infected you and to whom you may have passed this little goodie. No one will be penalized, but attempts will be made to ensure that everyone receives treatment. Also, sexually transmitted diseases are good bedfellows with one another, so testing for syphilis, chlamydia, and HIV is a good idea. Transmission of gonorrhea following a single sex act is 50 percent male to female, and 20 percent female to male.

Condoms—male or female—can prevent the spread of gonorrhea. It is also necessary for us to overcome shyness about these issues and talk frankly with our partners . . . and of course, it helps to know your partner for a while, although that is not always adequate insurance, as Emma's story demonstrates.

HERPES

Herpes is an extremely common condition worldwide and appears to be on the increase. It is equally common in all socioeconomic and racial groups, and in both developed and developing countries.

Dylan is a very handsome young man who prides himself on his physique. He works out daily and looks like an ad for fitness products. Dylan has worked in the travel industry ever since high school, when he helped out in his parents' travel agency. He has also been quite sexually active, in a very casual way, since he was sixteen.

When Dylan was twenty-three, shortly before he met his wife, Kathy, he had a little fling—or, to be precise, a one-night stand—with a girl he met at a party. They had both drunk quite a bit and she was on the Pill, so his usual caution was thrown to the wind and no protection was used. About a week later, he felt really under the weather, as though he was coming down with the flu. This passed, but then he noticed that he had a weird tingly, burning sensation in his penis. A few days later, blisters appeared on the skin of his penis, all along the shaft, and the lightbulb flashed.

Sure enough, the doctor told him he had herpes and gave him a prescription for acyclovir, explaining that the first episode is always the worst and the acyclovir would shorten it and decrease the severity. Even so, the blisters turned to ulcers that sort of ran together, his whole penis felt very raw and the glands in his groin were swollen and sore. He had just begun a new job as a travel representative with a major airline and hated to lose any work so soon, but had to take a week off because he couldn't walk— the pressure of his trousers was agonizing!

About three months later, Dylan had a second episode. This one was not half so bad. He had the mild tingling on the penis, but there were only a few blisters and ulcers. His glands didn't swell at all. This was a relief, because he was away overseas on business and couldn't afford to lose any time trying to find a doctor in a strange city. Six months later, he felt the tingling, went straight to his own doctor, started the acyclovir and nipped it in the bud.

It was around this time that he met Kathy. Within a month of starting dating, he realized that this was the woman he wanted to marry. He told her that he'd had a "little something" once, but that it had been treated and wasn't anything to worry about. They were using condoms religiously and he figured that she was safe.

After a year of serious dating, Kathy and Dylan moved in together. Kathy went on the Pill and they stopped using condoms. Dylan hadn't had an episode of herpes for so long that he figured he was cured.

After an additional episode-free year, the couple married and settled into a happy newlywed routine. All went well for another nine months—too well, perhaps, because Dylan received a big promotion in his job and started to work long hours and bring paperwork home. He was losing sleep and wasn't able to get to the gym every day. One Friday night, as he opened his front door, he suddenly felt that tingling again. Oh no! He sat Kathy down and embarked on a difficult recital—the "H" word hadn't ever really been mentioned before and now after so long . . . He could feel the freeze in the air as Kathy took in what he was saying. To make matters worse, it was too late to get to the doctor's that night so he had no professional ally to help tell her. He felt lower than dirt. The worst was still to come, though.

By Sunday, Kathy was running a fever and felt very ill. She couldn't even keep a bite of ice cream down. The next day, she experienced a painful burning and tingling at the vaginal opening and knew it had struck. She got in to see her family doctor the same morning, and received much sympathy, along with a prescription for acyclovir. Dr. Seip took the time to explain to her that this was a common affliction and that having it happen now didn't mean that Dylan had been cheating on her. She told Kathy that the virus, once acquired, resides in the cells beneath the skin and can remain latent for long periods of time and then be activated by stressors—in Dylan's case, probably the stress of his new position and the resultant fatigue. She also explained that the prescription should decrease the severity of this first attack, since Kathy was receiving it within the first six days.

By Wednesday, though, Kathy was totally incapacitated. Her vulva was covered with blisters and ulcers and the whole area was swollen. She couldn't do anything but lie in bed because she couldn't walk —any friction at all against her crotch caused a griping pain. Dylan turned into a nurse—in constant attendance, bringing cool compresses, aspirin, and a strong drink. He looked like a mournful dog with the shame of it all. He was also worrying that she'd never have sex with him again.

On Wednesday night they had to throw in the towel and go to the emergency room. Kathy couldn't pee. She was catheterized and admitted for IV fluids and pain medication. Dr. Seip suggested, when Kathy was sent home, that Kathy take acyclovir daily for at least a year to suppress the virus, because Kathy had had such a bad first episode. She also called the couple in to see her a week later and then discussed with them the ramifications of all this for their desire to start a family in the near future. She explained that if Kathy had an attack around the time her baby was due, she might have to have a caesarean to avoid the baby developing a serious infection, but that this was a safe procedure and no reason to decide against trying for a pregnancy.

Herpes can destroy relationships, but fortunately Kathy and Dylan had worked hard at talking through problems and had built a relationship based on honesty. Kathy believed Dylan that this was not a new infection and forgave his rather naïve neglect of openness about it. Dr. Seip was tremendously helpful to the young couple and helped them to see that this was not the end of the world and that they could still realize all their dreams.

Genital herpes is caused by herpes simplex, type 2. This is a virus and there are other members of the herpes virus family. Type 1 causes the common cold sore and, much less often than type 2, can also cause a genital herpes infection. But here, to all intents and purposes, we are not talking about type 1. Make no mistake about it: genital herpes is a sexually transmitted disease. You will not get it from using your friend's towel. The virus likes warm, moist areas and can infect the genitals, mouth, throat, and anus—in other words, wherever sexual contact may occur. Condoms can protect to a great extent but not completely, and the virus may be passed to a sexual partner even when no symptoms are present.

Within two to twenty days of exposure, you may experience—as did Dylan—flu-like symptoms, followed by tingling and pain. Dylan experienced this on his penis, but

DICK

it can occur anywhere in the lower pelvic area. Then come the blisters, which quickly open out to shallow and very painful ulcers. The active manifestation of the illness is self-limiting and the ulcers and pain clear within two weeks for most people. Each occurrence is usually milder than the last, with the first being the worst. Treatment helps to moderate the severity and length of the outbreak and is most effective in the first episode. As mentioned before, treatment needs to begin during the first six days of symptoms.

It is critical to understand that, although the rash goes away and the outbreaks get milder, the virus resides happily in your cells and you remain infected. Our drugs can suppress it (like caging a wild lion), but will not cure it. Therefore, if you have new sexual partners, you need to be honest with them. If you have an active attack, it is best to abstain from intercourse; otherwise, use condoms at all times. Although we are not sure that these measures are 100 percent effective, studies of monogamous couples in which one partner has the infection and the other doesn't indicate about a 15 percent infectivity over an eighteen-month period.

Herpes infection doesn't mean that you are dirty or promiscuous or a social leper. It means that you need to be careful and honest in your sexual relationships. Health care workers can help you explain to partners if any difficulty arises.

As we've intimated, the newborn baby is the greatest victim of genital herpes. There is about a 60 percent mortality rate associated with neonatal herpes infection. So it is important that doctors caring for pregnant women are informed if a woman and/or her partner has ever had genital herpes so that appropriate measures can be taken.

Some fortunate souls never have a recurrence after the initial attack of herpes, while others are plagued with frequent recurrences. The difference has nothing to do with virtue or lack thereof. We quite frankly don't understand why it acts like this, but need to accept that it does. Recurrences seem to correlate with times of greater stress, be it physical, emotional, or a combination, as in Dylan's case. Stress alters our immune responses, so this makes sense. Other illnesses obviously stress one's body greatly, and it is not uncommon for an attack of herpes to add to the discomfort of another illness.

This leads us to the association with HIV. While not yet cast in stone, there are clear indications in various studies that people with herpes simplex, type 2 are more susceptible to HIV when they are exposed to it. It is also known that herpes infection complicates HIV. We used to think that herpes posed an increased risk for cervical cancer, but we now know that the association is actually more with human papilloma virus, which we'll talk about later. The bottom line is that these STDs make good bedfellows for each other and, when one is diagnosed, the others should be tested for.

As we've mentioned, we can treat herpes infections with antiviral drugs, like acyclovir and valacyclovir, but these do not cure the infection—they only suppress the virus. Other treatments aimed at relieving the pain and discomfort are local cool compresses and oral or, more rarely, IV pain medication. Complementary medicine advocates the use of l-lysine, an amino acid, both to treat and prevent the attacks. It is further advocated that infected people avoid foods high in methionine, like nuts and seeds, because these interfere with lysine. Studies are lacking to confirm or deny the efficacy of this approach, but it is not harmful. Advocates use 500 milligrams of l-lysine three times daily when the virus is active and 500 milligrams daily otherwise.

GENITAL WARTS

Genital warts, caused by human papillomavirus, are probably the most common STD in the world at the present time, with millions of new infections every year. Despite this dramatic statistic, a number of studies assessing people's knowledge of the disease have indicated an alarming lack of information.

Before we get very far into this, let us assure you that common warts are just that—common, and they occur on the penis as well as elsewhere on the body.

The viruses that cause warts—common and genital (known as *Condyloma accuminata*)—live in the skin even when there is no visible sign of them. This is why warts often seem to pop up out of the blue.

Kylie was a college student spending a year overseas. She met Per, a real hunk of a Norwegian, on the train from Brussels to Rome—a long enough trip to get an acquaintance well established. In Rome, they enjoyed ten days of fabulous sex and sightseeing, then Kylie was off back home to her studies. Rome and Per were relegated to the happy memories category and routine took over.

A few months later, Kylie went to her local medical center for her annual Pap smear and pill prescription. Jocelyn, the women's health doctor, delivered the nasty news: "Kylie, you have genital warts here at the back of the vagina. I want to take a swab as well as your Pap smear and get confirmation of this and also have them typed because some types can predispose to cervical cancer."

Kylie kept calm until she was home in her bedroom and then, despite Jocelyn's reassurances, the tears flowed freely. Jocelyn had said that she'd phone in about a week to ten days but Kylie felt she couldn't bear the waiting. "God, what if I have cervical cancer at age twenty? What'll I do? I want kids. Mom and Dad will just die."

The week passed and Jocelyn phoned with the news that Kylie did indeed have genital warts, but they were not of the types that had strong associations with cervical (and penile) cancer, and that her Pap smear was normal. An appointment was made for Kylie to go in for treatment of the warts.

Kylie's story is not at all uncommon. We have seen genital warts on very young adolescents—if you are sexually active and not using condoms, you are at risk. When Jocelyn gently asked Kylie about condom use, she admitted she had been a little lax in that area.

There are at least a hundred different members of the human papillomavirus (HPV) family and about half of these choose the genital area (including the anus) as their preferred abode. They usually reside happily in the cells, remaining invisible. It is estimated that 20–40 percent of adults have at least one type of HPV residing in the cells in their genital area and that most of these people are completely free of any symptoms. This is why a woman can be shocked when a routine Pap smear comes back indicating the probability of HPV when she has never had any warts or suspicious bumps. Actually, visible warts only occur in about 10 percent of all HPV infections, and Per may have been unaware that he was affected.

The types of HPV most commonly associated with the development of cervical cancer (and cancer of the penis) are 16, 18 and 31. These are not usually associated with obvious genital warts but are usually diagnosed when the Pap smear indicates HPV is present and then typing is done. On the other hand, the most common types associated with obvious warts are types 6 and 11, and they are rarely, if ever, associated with cancer. So, you see, there is good news as well as bad.

In men, warts may appear on the penis, scrotum, buttocks, and around the anus. In women, they appear on the vulva and perineum, cervix, and anus. It is unusual to find them on the vaginal walls.

Genital swab tests are now available to check men and women for a myriad of STDs, including HPV. It is well worth having these tests done periodically if you are sexually active and not monogamous (and monogamous means you are *both* monogamous). We've given the depressing association of HPV with cervical cancer in women, but we need to emphasize now that surveillance with more frequent Pap smears and colposcopy can detect changes in the cervix while they are still precancerous and often lead to cure by localized intervention, such as diathermy, laser, or cryosurgery (freezing). It is likely that tests for viral typing will also become more common in the next few years. When the precancerous types of HPV are present, increased vigilance needs to persist throughout the woman's life and her partner needs to be aware of this too. There is also an increased risk of cancer of the penis and anus, when these are affected by HPV or visible warts, but it seems that neither of these is as common as cervical cancer is in women. Condoms consistently used give good, though not complete, protection. There is also the welcome news that a vaccine effective at preventing the high-risk HPV infections is on the horizon.

Treatment for genital warts used to involve repeated visits to the doctor's office to have them painted with podophyllin, a treatment associated with a lot of burning and discomfort, especially if it inadvertently got on to healthy skin. Podophyllin is no longer recommended for genital warts and we now have two drugs, podophyllo-toxin and imiquimod, which you can apply in the privacy of your home. These are safer and more effective. More extensive warts can sometimes be treated with freezing (cryotherapy) in your doctor's office. If you should be cursed with warts like Harry's, which looked like broccoli around his anus, you will need to have them surgically removed.

SYPHILIS

There are about twelve million new cases of syphilis per year reported throughout the world. This is depressing news considering that syphilis is very easily cured in its early stages by a cheap antibiotic, penicillin, and that the long-term effects of the disease can be devastating and often fatal.

Many historians consider syphilis a native American disease. Indisputable references to it in European history only occur after Columbus's return from the New World. However it got there, syphilis was rampant in sixteenth-century Europe and was known as the pox, French disease, or French pox. It was a democratic illness and crossed all socioeconomic and geographic borders. The preventive medicine of the day was to impose sanctions on prostitutes and to give various herbal possets.

Paracelsus incited the ire of the city fathers of Nuremburg in 1530 by writing a scholarly description of the symptoms of syphilis, and advocating the treatment of the illness by carefully calculated doses of mercury compounds. In this, he was centuries ahead of the mercury-based Salvarsan treatment of 1909. Salvarsan was the first successful drug treatment of syphilis. In 1943, during World War II, a breakthrough came. It was discovered that a one-week course of treatment with the brand-new drug penicillin cured syphilis.

There are two types of syphilis: acquired, which means that you pick it up yourself; and congenital, which means your parents gave it to you at birth by being infected themselves.

Syphilis has three stages and has been called the great mimic, because its symptoms are so diverse. In the first stage, which occurs anywhere from one to six weeks after exposure (sex with an affected person), there appears at the point of contact (penis, mouth, throat, anus) a small, hard, painless bump. This enlarges and ulcerates. This is called the chancre and, if seen, is diagnostic of primary syphilis. Its margins remain hard and raised and it is still painless. All too often, this chancre goes unnoticed.

One late and reasonably uneventful night in the emergency room, Michele was called to a cubicle where a young man sat upright on the examination table. He complained of a sore throat, but answered no to all the questions relating to cold symptoms, fever, runny nose, etc. As Michele shone the light into his throat to take a throat swab, she saw a classical syphilitic chancre winking at her from the man's tonsil. This changed things considerably!

If the chancre is not detected—and this is often the case when it is on the cervix and causes no other symptoms—it will heal and disappear within ten to forty days, leaving the person still infected.

The second stage of syphilis occurs after the chancre heals, and is characterized by many vague symptoms, including fever, joint symptoms, flu-like symptoms, and rashes on the skin and mucous membranes. These skin manifestations are highly contagious. All of these vague symptoms can persist, off and on, for many years. The rashes are the most easily recognizable signs of secondary syphilis and will lead a doctor to order confirmatory blood tests, although many sufferers are never diagnosed during this stage. The syphilis bugs then stay quietly in the body, moving on to the final, or tertiary, stage of syphilis, which develops within three to twenty-five years in about one-third of untreated syphilis patients. This stage can permanently affect the heart, blood vessels, brain, and nervous system, and may be fatal.

Syphilis is curable by antibiotics in the primary and secondary stages and the latent phase before the organ changes of the tertiary stage develop; these later changes are not reversible.

Phoebe was fifty-six years old and had a terrible bout of Bell's palsy, causing the left side of her face to droop. She was having trouble with her left eye and thought it was because of the palsy. To her horror and indignation, the ophthalmologist saw changes on her retina that led him to test her for syphilis and the tests were positive! The tragedy of it all is that Phoebe was an abused wife, whose very jealous second husband beat her for imaginary affairs. Somehow, he had to be tested and treated without making him in any way consider blaming her. The ophthalmologist handled it with exquisite tact and finesse.

Grace was a young woman having her first baby in a country hospital. She turned up to book with Caroline for the birth when she was fourteen weeks pregnant. A routine blood test showed that Grace was actively infected with syphilis, which could seriously harm her baby. She was given two shots of penicillin (one in each buttock, a week apart, definitely an ouch!) which cleared the infection before her baby was harmed. Grace's partner Eddy also came up positive for syphilis on blood tests and had the same penicillin shots.

Both of these women had caught syphilis from their infected partners, but had been unaware of their earlier infection. This is how most late syphilis is diagnosed: in women—medical screening in another context picks it up. We also recommend screening whenever another STD is diagnosed: as we've said, these little fellows often travel together . . .

Congenital syphilis is contracted by infection across the placenta—that is, an infected mother transmits the infection to her baby in the womb. This has now become very uncommon in the developed world, thanks to antenatal testing for syphilis and prompt treatment like Grace had.

CHLAMYDIA

Chlamydia is a most silent scourge: there are millions of new infections worldwide each year, but the infected often have no inkling of a problem until complications result. It is caused by a microscopic organism called *Chlamydia trachomatis* that has some properties of both bacteria and viruses. This organism is a delicate creature that does not readily survive outside the body; it is transmitted only by sexual contact. Its unique culture needs defied our ability to diagnose infection until the late 1970s. Even then, culture was not feasible unless the specimen was very quickly transported to a lab with the technical capabilities to perform these cultures; this effectively meant that diagnostic testing was not available in most rural areas.

George is a college student in a large university town. One morning, he experienced a terrible burning when he tried to pee. George was lucky; he went to the student health services and the doctor there did a swab from his urethra (which hurt like hell, he's quick to tell you) and within forty-eight hours had the news from the lab that he had chlamydia. Two weeks of a cheap antibiotic cleared it right up. Of course, the doctor also insisted that George contact the two young women students with whom he'd had sex in the previous two weeks, so they could be tested too. This was highly embarrassing for George, though he could see it was only right, and it had the effect of making him decide he'd always use condoms in the future.

Nonspecific or *non-gonococcal urethritis* is characterized by inflammation of the urethra, leading to burning on urination and sometimes a discharge from the penis. We know now that the vast majority of these cases are caused by chlamydia, as in George's case, but some may be due to other organisms. These cases also often respond to antibiotics. Unfortunately, there is a tendency for the symptoms of urethritis to recur, and occasionally for symptoms to appear elsewhere, including a combination of inflammation of the eyes (conjunctivitis), inflammation of the joints (arthritis), and skin rashes, especially on the feet. This little collection of goodies is called *Reiter's syndrome* and requires the ongoing care of a specialist physician—it is also yet another good reason to always use those condoms in the first place.

Many women never know that they have been infected with chlamydia until they need to investigate their inability to make babies. To avoid this situation, many doctors and clinics routinely screen young women for chlamydia. We now have simple swab and urine tests that rely on DNA typing. These have good accuracy and can easily be done at the same time as a Pap smear.

If chlamydia is detected on a routine screen, a course of antibiotics will cure it and prevent the complications of infertility. Follow-up testing to ensure it has cleared is also a good idea.

HEPATITIS B

Hepatitis B deserves its place among the STDs. Several million cases occur every year in both developed and undeveloped countries as a result of sexual transmission.

Hepatitis B is caused by a virus and is transmitted from one person to another by infected body secretions. Once infection occurs, the incubation period can be anywhere from four weeks to six months. However, a blood test may be positive as soon as two weeks after being exposed to the virus.

Hepatitis B is not an insignificant illness. Russell didn't know that he was infected until about four months after his marriage to Nell. They had been intimately involved for several years, but Russell had maintained other relationships with both men and women until shortly before their actual marriage. After finally coming to this decision, they had moved away from the "big city" to a more rural area, all primed for an idyllic life together. One weekend, Russell realized that he was feeling exceptionally tired—far more exhausted than a forty-year-old man should feel. Nell had just had a positive pregnancy test, so maybe it was psychological. But by Monday Russell knew that this was definitely not in his head—he felt awful. He had a low-grade fever, muscle aches, and extreme fatigue; he also had no appetite and could keep nothing down anyway. By Tuesday, his skin had a golden hue and his eyes looked yellow. It was time to see a doctor! Much to his surprise, Dr. Clarke hospitalized him. Within a few days, it was confirmed: not only did Russell have hepatitis, but it was hepatitis B. His recovery was slow and, even after he returned home, Russell didn't return to really feeling quite himself. Six months later, he received the daunting news that he now had chronic hepatitis—much more common with hepatitis B than other forms. By now, he was also a new father and the combination was almost more than he could bear. Not all our stories have happy endings: Russell died of liver cancer two days after his daughter entered kindergarten.

Russell's story illustrates the worst-case scenario of hepatitis B. The range can be from very mild illness—kind of like a stomach flu—all the way to acute liver failure from massive liver necrosis (death) or chronic active hepatitis and cancer, like Russell had.

Treatment of hepatitis B is primarily supportive: in the face of nausea and vomiting or diarrhea, it may be necessary to give the patient IV fluids to treat and prevent dehydration. Rest is imperative and the usual course of the illness is about three months. It is important that follow-up blood tests be done to ensure that the person has recovered and that the illness has not become chronic.

A carrier state of hepatitis B also exists. In this state, a person may be infectious but not themselves have the clinical illness of hepatitis.

We are very fortunate now to have a safe and effective vaccine for hepatitis B. In the sexual climate of today, in which few young people will have one sexual partner for life, immunization against hepatitis B makes lots of sense, not only from a public health point of view, but also as real protection for our young people. The current immunization guidelines call for primary immunization of children against hepatitis B at birth.

TRICHOMONIASIS

Trichomoniasis is a sexually transmitted disease that is a common cause of great discomfort to women, though much less often to men. The *trichomonad* is a one-celled parasite that colonizes the urethra in the male, usually causing few or no symptoms. Once in a while, it causes discomfort when peeing, but nothing like some of the bugs we've just discussed. And, just occasionally, it can cause a nasty and painful inflammation of the prostate gland, with pain deep at the base of the penis and fever. In women, "trich" causes a burning vaginal discharge, which is greenish in color and foul smelling. It can also cause a urethritis and, less commonly, inflammation of the bladder.

Treatment is a course of Flagyl (metronidazole), an antibiotic. This is very effective, and we have not found alternatives to be very helpful. Both partners should be treated. Trichomoniasis is not usually associated with any long-term complications.

HIV

Darryl liked the ladies a lot—any lady, anywhere. Darryl had signed on with the Army and was away for six months on overseas duty. In accordance with the rules of supply and demand, ladies were plentiful near the base and his wick was well-tended; with time, Darryl grew careless about using protection and some of the women he went with did not insist. Darryl didn't think you could really catch HIV from a woman, so he didn't worry until the day he looked at his favorite part and noticed a wart on it.

He went to the infirmary and the doctor on duty suggested a full STD screen. "You have a genital wart there, Darryl, and in itself it's not that serious, but we'd better check for its partners in crime."

Three days later, Darryl was called to the infirmary and the doctor informed him that he was HIV positive.

Most people today have heard a lot about HIV/AIDS, but misconceptions linger. Let us give you an accurate outline of what HIV really means.

First of all, each and every act of intercourse has the potential for HIV exposure. We, in medicine, practice what we call universal precautions: this means that we don't try to second-guess the risks: we treat each patient encounter as a potential for infectious exposure and we use all the barriers necessary and possible to prevent disease transmission. In our case, this means gloves, goggles, and similar equipment; in yours, it means condoms.

Second, AIDS is caused by HIV. There are a number of strains of the virus and this fact, together with sexual habits, explains why heterosexual spread is less in some countries and unfortunately so common in a number of others. Homosexual transmission happens in all countries. But don't fool yourself by thinking that heterosexual sex is free of HIV risk: it is definitely not.

Third, while HIV/AIDS can be treated by a variety of drugs, this is management, not cure. Prevention is the only known cure and safe sex is still the only effective preventive measure available. Obviously, abstinence is the safest sex unless you are in a committed monogamous relationship. We have no vaccine at this time.

These are facts, not moral judgments or prudery. AIDS is currently as great a threat to the survival of many populations as war.

And what happened to Darryl? Darryl's doc counseled

him well and told him that he was infected with the virus but didn't yet have AIDS . . . this would require careful and diligent monitoring of his viral load to be aware of when the viral count began to rise in order to start medications.

Although some people may have a flu-like illness within a month or two of exposure to the virus, Darryl had no symptoms. He was warned to watch for such an illness, with symptoms of fever, headache, general malaise, and swelling of his lymph glands, most easily felt in the neck and groin. He was warned that, whether he developed symptoms or remained asymptomatic for months or years, he was still highly infectious and would have to rethink his play style. He was told that, as the virus disabled and killed the cells of his immune system, he would gradually have less resistance to common infections, may develop yeast infections, and would eventually lose weight, have bad headaches, cough, be extremely fatigued, and have symptoms such as shortness of breath, depending upon which organs were affected. Certain cancers, such as Kaposi's sarcoma, would also then become more likely. Not a good scenario.

Fortunately, since Darryl was diagnosed early, he would benefit from a "drug cocktail" regimen that would keep his viral load down and help to prolong his life and maintain its quality. The combinations of drugs available and used are too complex and too constantly evolving for us to go into them here. Darryl was encouraged but also warned that these did not constitute a cure, but merely disease management.

Today, Darryl has left the army and is working at an office job. He has married a lovely woman, Marla, a nurse

<sub>who understands Darryl's situation well. They practice safe
sex and have thought about adopting children but decided
against it because of the uncertainty of Darryl's future.</sub>

Darryl was both lucky and unlucky—his luck in all of
this came from his early diagnosis. Although our biggest
message to you is "safe sex," the secondary message should
be to have a screening for STDs, including HIV, every six
to twelve months if you are active with multiple partners.
And remember: age has nothing to do with this. After all,
the combination of Viagra and prostitution has led to a rise
in HIV amongst senior citizens in Miami, Florida!

LESS COMMON STDS

Granuloma inguinale (Donovanosis)

Although relatively uncommon in temperate climates,
Granuloma inguinale is worth at least a brief discussion, as it
is common in the tropics.

James was in the Air Force, stationed in the Southwest
Pacific. On leave, he flew to the Philippines for a little
"R&R." During his first six hours in Manila, he met a
gorgeous woman in the hotel lounge. The next forty-eight
hours were a blur of partying and sex, and then it was back
to the base. It was all a very pleasant memory until, a little
more than two months later, he noticed a hard pimple-like
thing on his joy stick. It didn't hurt so he ignored it for a
week or so, then he noticed that it was marking his jockeys
with a yellow stain. It also seemed to be spreading and
getting bigger. There were also some tiny painless lumps
in his groin. At this point, he decided a trip to the
squadron's doctor would be smart.

The doctor took scrapings and swabs from the sore and

did lots of blood tests. He told James he was pretty sure that it was *Granuloma inguinale*, but he'd check for all the STDs just to be sure. He then proceeded to give James the lecture of his life on always using protection, taking his common sense along on leave, and other advice along these lines, after which he sent him off to take antibiotics for two weeks.

The risk of contracting *Granuloma inguinale*, like all STDs, is increased with multiple sexual partners, visiting prostitutes, and unprotected sex. The initial sore can become infected with other bugs, giving a very unpleasant bad-smelling discharge. *Granuloma inguinale*, or Donovanosis as it's also called, is common in Northern Australia, and even more so in Papua New Guinea, as well as other Pacific and Southeast Asian countries. Fortunately the bug is sensitive to several good antibiotics—it's important to take the full course.

Chancroid

Chancroid is characterized by painful, oozing ulcers, preceded by small, painful pimple-like lesions, and accompanied by swelling of the lymph glands. It is most commonly confused with herpes when patients first notice it, and may also be confused with the skin changes of syphilis. Obviously it is important that ulcers on Dick or in the surrounding area are properly diagnosed, so that the correct treatment and prognosis can be given. Unlike herpes, chancroid is curable by antibiotic treatment.

Just to mention it one more time: the big take-home message from all these stories is the need to practice safe sex, whether vaginal, oral or anal. No, it's not a 100 percent guarantee against picking up any of these bugs but it's the best prevention we have right now.

151

It was a man, not a woman—in fact, the actor Robin Williams—who said that God gave men a brain and a penis but not enough blood to run both at the same time. We think that in fact it is possible! Yes, safe sex requires some thought and preparation, but the payoff, as you can see from our stories, is definitely worth it.

NON-SEXUALLY TRANSMITTED INFECTIOUS DISEASES OF THE PENIS

Candida

Candida, or *thrush*, is the cause of a great deal of recurring discomfort in women, and may be passed between sexual partners, but is not really considered a sexually transmitted disease. A man may get a "yeast" infection on the glans of his penis after having sex with an infected woman, but he is unlikely to pass this to further partners and it is usually readily treated by antifungal creams. A woman who is bothered by recurrent infections may be asked by her doctor to get her partner to apply one of these creams to the glans and shaft of his penis—this simply stops the poor woman becoming reinfected, and there are no underlying implications. Both men and women will often get fungal infections in the groin or other warm, moist areas; it is a common problem. In those who need to wear diapers or other incontinence protection, thrush can be annoyingly persistent. Antifungal creams and ointments that protect the skin from moisture, such as zinc oxide, are very helpful.

The penis is well supplied with tiny glands and folli- cles whose purpose is the secretion of lubrication of the skin and mucous membranes. These can become infected by a number of organisms, especially when hygiene is poor. Often, topical cleansing, warm packs, and topical antibiotics are all that are necessary to heal these. If pain, redness, or itching continue, consult your doctor.

The testes, epididymis, and scrotum are not immune to infectious illness. Tuberculosis (TB) is a pestilence that is again on the rise; as a result, we will undoubtedly again be seeing tuberculous infections of the testes and/or epididymis. Indeed, in many parts of the world, TB is the most prevalent health problem and is closely allied with HIV infection.

Mumps

Prior to widespread immunization of preschool children against mumps, *orchitis*—or inflammation of the testes due to mumps—happened in about a quarter of all adolescents and young men who had mumps. It is uncommon in boys who have mumps at a younger age. Of course, today mumps is rarely seen, thanks to immunization. When it does occur in teenage boys or older men, it may cause severe pain and swelling of the testes, with subsequent atrophy or shrinking associated with reduced or absent fertility.

Filariasis

The world has shrunk in the past decade. Globalization of trade has sent professional people thousands of miles from their home bases and, in the process, has exposed them to illnesses they've never heard of. *Elephantiasis*, or filariasis, caused by *Wucheria bancrofti*, a parasite spread to humans by mosquito bites, causes huge swelling of the scrotum and the skin of the penis. This is typically a tropical disease, but travelers from temperate zones are not immune. This is not a happy way to get a big dick! The best prevention is careful protection against mosquito bites when visiting affected areas of the world.

Urinary tract infection

While the infection here is more in the bladder, kidneys, and ureters (the tubes that connect the kidneys and bladder), Dick is certainly involved, so we'll talk a little about urinary tract infection (UTI) at this point. UTI is not nearly as common in men and boys as in women and girls but it does still occur (the reason for the difference, as you can quickly understand, is the much greater length of the male urethra, which makes it harder for the bugs causing the infection to actually make their way up into the bladder). One exception is in newborn babies. Little boys who have not been circumcised are more likely to get UTIs than those who've had their tiny foreskins chopped off. As we've explained though, these infections are not sufficient cause to justify the procedure of circumcision, and will respond to antibiotics.

The bugs that cause UTI are generally those living happily and normally in the bowel or on the skin of the genital region. One way or another—by traveling up the urethra or in the bloodstream—they get into the bladder, take up residence and multiply, and may spread farther upward to the ureters and kidneys, causing severe infections if untreated.

In babies and little boys, the signs of UTI may be non-specific—they may have a loss of appetite, vomiting, and hot, rather than having any obvious tummy pains or burning while urinating. Older boys are more likely to have definite complaints, same as in adults—it hurts to pee, they need to pee more often, and there may be pain and tenderness over the lower abdomen and the middle of the back (over the kidneys).

Urinary tract infection is diagnosed by growing the bugs in the laboratory after obtaining a clean catch specimen of urine or a midstream urine, to avoid contamination from skin contact. The lab also tests the sensitivity of the bugs to various antibiotics so that the right treatment can be given. Antibiotic courses should always be completed even though the pain and burning disappear quickly, otherwise the infection may recur.

In young children, UTI is often related to some abnormality in the anatomy of the bladder or kidneys so it is a good idea to check this out in any boy who has had a proven UTI—usually with a simple ultrasound examination. One common finding is backflow from the bladder into the ureters because the valves that should prevent this aren't working properly. This condition can be treated, but details of this are beyond the scope of our book—such children are cared for by specialist urologists.

In men of middle age and beyond, UTI may be related to enlargement of the prostate gland. As we mentioned in Chapter 11, benign enlargement of the prostate gland is extremely common in Caucasian men over fifty, less so in men of Asian origin and rare in black men. A well-known nineteenth-century surgeon named Benjamin Brodie remarked that "when the hair becomes grey and scanty, and specks of earthy matter become deposited in the arteries . . . the prostate gland, I might perhaps say invariably, becomes increased in size." The enlarged prostate, pressing on the urethra that runs through it, will cause urine to stagnate in the bladder, predisposing to infection.

Throughout this chapter, we have discussed the fact that diagnosis of the various infectious diseases needs to be done by a trained professional and that often laboratory tests are needed. Some diseases are sexually transmitted, some are not. Don't assume that there has been hanky-panky—go and get a diagnosis. You can figure the rest out later ... after treatment.

INFERTILITY: "IT'S JUST NOT HAPPENING" 18

The urge to perpetuate oneself by having children is basic to many people. About 85 percent of couples trying to conceive, using no birth control methods and having regular sexual intercourse, will achieve a pregnancy within a year. By definition, the remaining 15 percent have some kind of problem with fertility.

Sometimes the reason for this is obvious: Anthony and Katarina consulted Caroline because they had been married for eight months and were very anxious to have a baby. Anthony and Katarina both come from very religious backgrounds, were virgins when they married and were sexually very naïve. In talking with them, it was soon evident that they had never had full sexual intercourse. Surprising, you may think, in today's free-and-easy climate, but it does still happen. Caroline found that Anthony's tendency to premature ejaculation and Katarina's rather thick hymen (membrane across the vaginal opening), taken together, meant that sperm weren't getting anywhere near where they should be. What's more, neither partner was enjoying it much.

So the first (and often overlooked) question is: are you having sex with vaginal penetration by the penis and ejaculation of semen into the upper part of the vagina? If you are not, then that is the first step. And we're not being trite when we say that Nature intended it to be fun! If you need help or advice about sexual technique or problems, it is available from people who are trained and sympathetic—either talk to your family doctor, or see the suggestions at the end of this book.

You also need to be "doing it" at the right time of the month, as Kiri and Alf found.

Kiri's cycle was always regular at twenty-eight days, but when her doctor checked that she was ovulating, it became apparent that Kiri always ovulated midweek. Now this wouldn't be a problem except that Alf was never home midweek—he drives trucks and was gone from Monday to Friday. Sperm survive about seventy-two hours, and the egg is ready for fertilization for about twelve hours, so by Friday evening of the week that Kiri ovulated it was just too late. Kiri came up with a clever solution: she took the week off from her shop job and went with Alf. "It was a vacation with a difference!" she said. It worked. Little Tess was born nine months after her parents' trucking honeymoon.

If you have conscientiously tried the above methods, and no pregnancy has resulted, then you need to consider investigation and maybe treatment. We think it's worth pointing out that this is a good time for both partners to talk frankly with each other about their expectations. Very sophisticated technology is now available to treat many causes of infertility. But success rates for some of these procedures are nowhere near 100 percent. Today, more couples are also choosing to remain childless. This is a perfectly reasonable choice. Having tried for a while to conceive, and not succeeded, you both might decide not to pursue investigations. It is important, though, that any decision be mutual. If you are going to proceed, have some idea how far you want to go. Infertility treatments can be expensive, time-consuming, painful, and in some cases risky, as well as possibly unsuccessful. Having some endpoint in mind from the beginning is a sensible plan.

Studies have indicated that, in approximately 30 percent of infertility cases, the cause is in the man alone and, in another 20 percent, both partners have a problem preventing pregnancy. So the bottom line is that the man is implicated at least 50 percent of the time.

Any investigation of infertility should regard the couple as a unit. Kevin came in to Michele's office for an insurance physical and said: "Oh, by the way, Doc, Nora and I have wanted a baby for a long time and nothing is happening." He could think of nothing significant in his medical past and "everything works fine, Doc." However, on examining him, Kevin had some interesting findings. He had a very light beard, which he attributed to being blond, and his body hair growth was scanty. He also had genital development that looked like it had gotten stuck at early adolescence. Clearly, there was a possible problem here. However, when Michele tried to tell Kevin about this and suggest further investigations, he became most embarrassed and refused to consider it any further. He also declined bringing Nora into the discussion, so investigations could not proceed.

The initial evaluation of infertility involves a good history from both partners, including questions related to health, sexual habits, social habits, and other symptoms, because these all give us clues as to what might be going on. Next, a good general medical examination should be performed for both of you. Your family doctor or another general practitioner or family planning clinic doctor is the best person to do this—you don't need specialist input at this stage.

Clearly, if some gynecological problem is detected, this will need investigation and maybe referral to a gynecologist; this is beyond the scope of this book. If a medical problem is known or detected in the male partner, this too will need attention. However, regardless of both of these possibilities, a sperm count and analysis of the semen will usually be indicated at this point.

Oh oh, we hear you say—believe us, guys, this is much simpler and less painful than most of the things your wife or partner will need to go through in the course of an infertility workup! There is absolutely no cause for embarrassment—laboratories are doing dozens of these tests every day: it's just routine for them.

Having a seminal analysis involves ejaculating into a cup provided by the laboratory, which can be done at home, or in a private room in a doctor's office, and getting the specimen to the lab as soon as possible so it can be looked at under the microscope. Most labs want it within two hours of production. Why the rush? Because we are concerned to know not only how many sperm there are, but also how motile they are—how well they can swim and thus find their way through the uterus to the Fallopian tubes where there is a hopeful egg waiting to be fertilized. You can produce your specimen by masturbation, by yourself or with your partner, or by starting to have intercourse and withdrawing before coming so that you come into the cup. It is important that all the semen from one ejaculation ends up in the cup.

It's a good idea to abstain from sex for a day or so before producing your semen sample.

If the first sample you produce fits easily into the parameters shown in Table 17.1, you won't need to produce any more. But a low sperm count, lowered motility, or other abnormality simply means that the test needs to be repeated—often more than once. Repeated tests are often normal. Even a persistent abnormality does not mean that pregnancy is impossible—only if you consistently show *no* sperm at all (what's called azoospermia) should a doctor tell you that you are not going to be able to father a child.

A detailed discussion of the causes of male infertility

Table 17.1 lists the details of a normal sample of semen and sperm count

normal semen volume 1 to 4 cc.
normal concentration of sperm 40 million per ml or greater
borderline 20 million per ml.
low less than 20 million per ml.
total sperm number >50 million
Motility = or > 50%   80% of sperm should have normal appearance

and sub-fertility is beyond the scope of this book, but we will try to categorize most of them. We've already seen that actually having intercourse and doing so at the right time is necessary to conception, so we'll omit that. But it is crucial.

Other factors can include:

- congenital problems, like chromosomal abnormalities (these are rare);
- hormonal problems—sometimes congenital, sometimes acquired;
- illnesses, including mumps, cirrhosis of the liver, kidney failure, sickle-cell disease, myotonic dystrophy, and several others;
- hemochromatosis—about 80 percent of men with this condition have some degree of testicular malfunction;
- the use of some drugs, especially steroids or other hormones;
- radiation;
- trauma to the testes or penis;
- undescended testes;
- scrotal varicocoele; and
- sperm disorders.

We'll discuss these briefly—obviously if you seem to have a problem with any of them, we would recommend you see a doctor who is competent to sort out what is going on and what to do about it.

Klinefelter's syndrome is the most common chromosomal anomaly and occurs once in about every five hundred men. It involves an extra X chromosome. We suspect Kevin has Klinefelter's sydrome—he certainly has the typical physical characteristics. Infertility in these men, which is due to the development of fibrous tissue and thickening within the testes, may be treatable, but other rarer chromosomal anomalies usually cause irreversible infertility.

There are a number of congenital conditions, often running in families, that cause hormonal problems. One of these is *Kallmann's syndrome*, which is the second most common cause of retarded development of the testes. That does not mean that it is common—it occurs in only one in 10,000 men. With Kallmann's syndrome, the pituitary hormones that stimulate the testes to produce its hormones and start sperm production are lacking.

Disease of the thyroid gland can affect sperm production. Problems such as tumors, or disease or trauma affecting the thyroid, adrenal or pituitary glands, can all have an adverse effect on the complicated process of producing healthy, active sperm that we described for you in Chapter 3. Most of these problems can be solved using artificial hormones to restore the hypothalamic–pituitary–testes pathway outlined in that chapter, so that the testes start to function normally again.

Taking hormones, like the anabolic steroids used illicitly by athletes, can also throw all these delicate mechanisms off-kilter. Unfortunately, so can the use of hormone drugs like Prednisone, which have made life much easier for some people with diseases like rheumatoid arthritis. Clearly, the solution in all these instances—if there is one—involves specialist care.

In the case of illness, the remedies are specific to the particular problem, and that needs a good medical definition. With the introduction of the mumps vaccine, we see fewer cases of mumps, *orchitis* (inflammation of those little orchids, the testes), than we used to, and therefore less infertility due to this, but it does still occur.

Hemochromatosis is an interesting illness. It is one of the more common inherited illnesses in Western countries and involves an abnormal deposit of iron in the tissues of the body. Eighty percent of men with hemochromatosis have some degree of fertility difficulty. It is hypothesized that deposits of iron in the testes interfere with the formation of healthy sperm.

Some drugs interfere with sperm production. Obviously some cancer drugs may do so (ask your doctor about your particular situation), but so may some commonly used drugs like the stomach drug cimetidine, the high blood pressure drug spironolactone, the antifungal ketoconazole, and salazopyrin, used for arthritis and inflammatory bowel disease. Check out any drugs you are taking with your doctor if you are concerned about fertility. Exposure to some pesticides and other chemicals may also have adverse effects on sperm.

Certain recreational drugs, such as marijuana, methadone, and heroin, may reduce testosterone levels. When Cora realized that Josh's dope habit might be keeping them from having children, there was a family explosion, resulting in all the weed paraphernalia ending up in the garbage. (The film *The Good Girl*, with Jennifer Aniston, hints at this!) Heavy alcohol consumption can also interfere with sperm production, and may reduce libido as well.

Radiation, whether for medical purposes or due to occupational exposure or an accident, can harm the very sensitive cells that form sperm. This is why the family jewels are always covered by a lead apron when you have an X-ray.

Obviously, the "balls" and penis are just hanging around, vulnerable to all kinds of trauma. It can be either quick and severe, such as a golf ball or a foot to the groin, or the repeated minor trauma of a cyclist training for a race. Hence the existence of athletic cups and jock straps for keeping Dick safe and sound and ready for later procreation. A history of an earlier injury, especially a large bruise (hematoma) of the scrotum, or a story of torsion of the testis (for more about these see Chapter 19) may provide clues as to why pregnancy is not happening.

Undescended testes are a common developmental defect, with an incidence of 0.8 percent in adult males. After about age two, the testes can no longer function normally in this condition; this is why pediatricians check the testes frequently in infants to pick up on this problem. It is important to repair this by surgically bringing the testes down into the scrotum both to preserve reproductive capacity and because there is a greater risk of testicular cancer in the undescended testis (more about this in Chapter 20).

Scrotal varicocoele (varicose veins in the scrotum) is the most common cause of male infertility found after investigation. (We both remember one of our teachers, a delightful and venerable Irish surgeon, demonstrating a varicocoele to us as medical students and saying "It feels like a bag of worms, doctor!") New diagnostic tools have indicated that up to 20 per cent of all men have a varicocoele. Amongst men presenting for infertility investigation, the incidence is closer to 50 percent.

The most common explanation for varicocoele-related infertility is that the raising of the testicular temperature and interference with blood flow by the varicose veins prevents good sperm production. However, only about 50 percent of men with a varicocoele have low sperm counts or other abnormalities when their semen is examined, so clearly this is not the whole story. It is common to do surgery—much like the surgery done for varicose veins in the legs—if an infertile man has a varicocoele. This surgery increases the chances of pregnancy, but may not be the whole bag of tricks.

> Dan is a career diplomat. He and Marie-Josephe had a fairy-tale romance when he met her while posted to her homeland of Senegal. They returned for a time to Dan's home in the United States and tried for the remainder of the following year to get pregnant, with no success. Dan's old family physician and long-time friend discovered that Dan had a varicocoele. Soon after Dan's surgery, he and Marie-Josephe were posted back to Senegal. Within two months, the pregnancy test was positive. And in duplicate—they were parents of twins within the year!

As we've mentioned, a good sperm needs to be healthy, with the right inner constituents and number of chromosomes; it also needs to be motile and able to penetrate the egg. This sounds simple enough, but in practice many little things can go awry.

Diagnosing and treating problems of sperm production are part of a highly specialized branch of medicine. If the sperm seem to be low in number or just not as active as is usual, they can nevertheless be helped to effect fertilization with technologies such as artificial insemination, invitro fertilization (IVF), or intracytoplasmic sperm injection (ICSI). Intracytoplasmic sperm injection involves obtaining a sample of sperm either by ejaculation or by sucking it out using a needle directed into the testis or epididymis (ouch! yes some local anesthetic is administered first). The latter procedure is done when there are obstructive problems in the tubes bringing the sperm from the testes to the penis, although the sperm themselves are normal enough to fertilize an egg successfully. It is also done in cases of retrograde ejaculation, where sperm "backfire," entering the bladder instead of passing into the urethra (this condition is discussed in Chapter 16).

Once the sperm are obtained, they are injected directly into the egg (which obviously also needs to be harvested from the woman) in the lab. This is the ICSI part of the procedure. Then the fertilized egg will be implanted in the woman's uterus. This is also a critically timed event, coordinated with the woman's cycle to ensure fertilization and subsequent implantation in the uterus. Most centers performing these sophisticated procedures report pregnancy rates of about 30 percent. In the case of those couples for whom they don't work, artificial insemination using donated sperm from a sperm bank is a possibility. You will need careful counseling and lots of discussion with your partner before deciding on this, since the child conceived will biologically have another father. Adoption and fostering are alternatives that may also be considered.

Jack and Rena had a combination problem—very low sperm counts on Jack's part and an irregular cycle on Rena's. After much thought, they decided to try ICSI and IVF. It worked and they conceived immediately. However, at eight weeks Rena had a miscarriage and the young couple were truly devastated. They didn't think they could ever go through this again, but after six months they decided to give it one more go . . . they now have a daughter who they named Prosperity, joking that she was such an investment.

On the other hand, April and Fergus, who had similar problems, looked at the cost of it all and decided to go with adoption, thinking that it would be more of a sure thing.

As you've undoubtedly realized by now, the investigation of infertility involves a medical history and physical exam, an analysis of the semen, and then any specialized blood tests, X-rays, or ultrasounds that the doctor thinks may help elucidate the cause of your problem, before any remedies are embarked upon. Any illnesses that are present (e.g. thyroid problems, diabetes) need to be treated and hormonal problems appropriately addressed. Although all of this is good for your health, it does not come with any cast-iron guarantee of a baby at the end of it. In around 30 percent of infertility cases, no obvious cause can be found in either partner and it is this "unexplained" group that has the lowest success rates from IVF and other technologies.

INJURIES: "WHAM, BAM—NO THANKS MA'AM"

19

(Be warned: This chapter contains low-level violence, and may get a little uncomfortable. Guys may want to keep a hand on their old jock straps or athletic cups before reading on.)

The good news is that trauma to Dick is actually not very common. This is largely due to how mobile, flexible and well-protected the penis is in its flaccid state. But when it does happen . . . oh my.

A friend of ours, a doctor named Pete, has given us permission to tell his story. We are indebted to him for this very personal account . . . it gives a whole new meaning to using a belt sander.

Pete and his partner Jess live in a very beautiful part of the world. They have been building their house over the past couple of years on a site overlooking a lovely lake. Pete works on it on his days off, and one sunny afternoon just before Christmas, Pete found himself on his own. Jess was off shopping and he thought he'd sand a large piece of mango wood that he was making into a table as a Christmas gift for her. It was going to be a showpiece in their dining room.

It was very hot and Pete was soon stripped down to nothing but a pair of shorts. He worked diligently for a couple of hours and was just thinking of stopping for a beer and bit of a relax, when "EEeeeeeeeeeeeeeeeeee." A searing pain shot from his groin to his fingertips and the sander made a strange groan and stopped. To his horror, Pete saw that his shorts and the end of Old Jack had disappeared into the minuscule space between the belt and the back of the sander—a space big enough to accommodate only a breath of air. To add to the injury, he could *smell* his own flesh and pubic hair burning.

Trying to keep a cool head, Pete assessed the situation: he would have to turn off the sander . . . and the power point was a good twenty feet away! Balancing the four and a half pound sander you-know-where, with gripping pain, he managed to get across the room and pull the cord. OK, so now he was safe from frying, but how could he get his best friend free from the #**#ing sander? If he couldn't get it off he'd have to drive the twenty minutes to the hospital balancing the sander on his old fella (or what might be left of it) and still keep from passing out. Not a good option. He did manage to get his fishing knife free from the tool box and cut the belt. As the blood rushed back into the mangled member, Pete was by this time lying on the floor. "All I could see were black and white trees, dim grey lake, all swaying gently in the bright afternoon sun. Swaying a lot, actually."

Just at this moment, Jess returned home and rushed Pete to the hospital where the hastily summoned plastic surgeon described it as "a particularly nasty injury." However, very fortunately the damage was confined to the skin. The corpora and large blood vessels remained intact. All the damaged skin had to be surgically removed and Pete underwent a series of skin grafts using skin from his thigh. "It's just as well I hadn't been circumcised as a kid," Pete said. "It left some room to maneuver. But I never thought I'd be circumcised by a sander."

Pete's injury was both an avulsing injury and a burn. Avulsing injury is the most common type of injury to Dick, and usually happens much as Pete described. Often such accidents occur in the course of working with industrial or farm machinery when loose clothing and the skin of the penis are caught in the machinery and skin gets pulled off. Obviously, these injuries vary from mild (a bit of foreskin) to severe (amputation of the whole penis).

In repairing any avulsing injury, all the skin and foreskin from the injury up to the glans needs to be surgically removed and replaced by a skin graft to prevent a permanent bumpy swelling at the end of the penis. If damage has occurred to blood vessels, i.e. the urethra and/or the spongy corpora, then expert microsurgery is needed. When part or all of the penis is irretrievably damaged or has to be amputated because it is beyond repair, subsequent plastic surgery using skin grafts and a prosthesis can restore the shape and appearance of Dick and, to a certain extent, the function. Clearly this is highly specialized surgery requiring both urologists and plastic surgeons and way beyond the scope of our book.

Pete tells us that, apart from the post-op pain, the most difficult part of recovery was avoiding thoughts of sex—or any stimulus that would give him an erection. Getting hard, even minimally so, brought exquisite pain. "For someone used to thinking of sex 634 times a day, like the average man, this was *not* fun. I instructed Jess not to wear her lacy underwear and bought her a vibrator—for some reason, I chose a model in virginal white. And of course I was worried whether the old guy would eventually perform like he used to. We had been planning to try for a pregnancy once the house was finished." Pete celebrated that Christmas flat on his back on the couch trying to divert his mind by watching TV.

Pete's story has a happy ending, though. He and Jess finished their house and last Christmas were gifted by the birth of a son, Hamish. Pete offers this advice: "Keep *all* your tools in good working order and never take your eyes off them. Maybe wearing a cup is a good idea when working with power tools."

Direct injuries to the penis, such as stab or bullet wounds, or crush injuries, are less common than avulsion or burns but obviously require urgent medical attention. And we'll just mention here a recent report from Sweden, of the professor who was seated (fully clothed) using his laptop literally on his lap, and who subsequently developed painful burns and blisters on his ivory pillar. Thankfully these cleared up without the need for surgery, but we would note that the makers of laptops do caution users against working on their devices while the base of the computer is against bare skin . . .

Another mechanism of injury involves rings or bands constricting the penis. In babies, this is not uncommonly caused by a hair—often the mother's—that somehow gets wrapped around the penis, causing swelling and making it impossible to see the hair. As we have mentioned, one of the approaches to a limp biscuit is a ring around the base of the penis so that the erection can't flop. This can be dangerous unless the ring is designed in a way that makes it very easy to release. Constriction causes swelling that makes it difficult to release the constriction and can compromise the blood supply to the penis. Get medical help, put ice on the penis, and hold it up until it is in the hands of an expert.

Almost every man has experienced the zipper injury. You know it well: you really have to take a leak badly and you pull the zip and nick yourself. Or you have the experience Craig had with Meghan. They were at it hot and heavy and Craig had slipped Meghan's silky things to the floor. His bazooka was bursting to get out and he yanked the zip. Immediately all thoughts of sex went out the window—and it didn't help that Meghan was immediately convulsed with laughter. The shrinkage freed him (it usually does), but if you find yourself in a bind, a little Vaseline or KY jelly will go a long way. Occasionally a visit to the emergency room is needed (don't be embarrassed, they've seen it all before), where local anesthetic may be needed before the skin is cut free; rarely does circumcision have to be performed.

Her fellow residents in her small country town still tell the story of Granny Jones who foiled a rapist by breaking his penis. We're not sure whether Granny did this deliberately or if it was just a result of her defensive efforts, but the upshot was the same—the rapist who had terrorized the women of the town for several months was stopped. Here's how she tells it: "He entered my house through the back window after I'd gone to bed and I awakened to find someone holding me down and ripping my nightie. I'd read the papers and knew what I was in for. He knocked me around but never hit me hard enough for me to lose consciousness and then he was banging away at me and it hurt. I gave my body a quick twist, mostly to try to protect myself and the next thing I knew, he collapsed across me and was making this high, keening sound. He was limp as a baby and I just hit my Lifeline button (you know, the one us old ones have in case we fall or something) and before he could regain his strength, the cops and ambulance were there and he was caught!"

Now, we've already told you that there are no bones in the penis, so you may be wondering what "broke." The cylinders of the corpora cavernosa are each encased in a membrane that stretches thin when they engorge with blood during erection. With a sharp blow or cutting injury of some type, this membrane can be torn or "broken." It can also happen with abnormal bending of the penis while it is erect.

The most common way for this to happen is during intercourse when the penis partly slips out of the vagina (or the woman twists, as Granny did) and then strikes the bony part of the woman's pelvis. This more commonly happens with the woman in the dominant position.

(The French—of course!—have a special name for this: *faux pas de coït*, which roughly translates as "a sexual stumble." *Oui*, indeed.) Other causes can be masturbation, industrial accidents (though why would you have a hard-on at work?), turning in bed with an erect penis, or any other movement that can give a quick abnormal flex to it.

This is a relatively uncommon injury, but is a surgical emergency when it happens. If you should be unfortunate enough to have it happen to you, we'd advise cold compresses and anti-inflammatory medications while getting to the emergency room as soon as possible. The aims in surgical treatment are to get rid of the blood clot and repair the membranes and any injury there may be to the urethra. In about eight weeks, the organ is again ready for action (though not, we are pleased to report, in the case of Granny's assailant, who is serving seven years).

This is probably the spot to emphasize the importance of protective gear for all athletic sports where Dick and/or his bag of tricks risk damage.

Ranjit was one of the best lacrosse players in the school. One day he was asked to fill in for a match at short notice; he was able to borrow a helmet, but didn't have a jock strap. He thought it wouldn't matter, and was playing defense, about to make an easy catch, when Owaaaaaaach! The ball hit the ground and so did Ranjit, with a huge bruise rapidly developing in his scrotum that needed to be aspirated with a needle that night in the emergency room. Worse, his painful walk around the school for several weeks afterwards had his friends doubled up with laughter. (We've already mentioned, too, that

occasionally damage like this can cause atrophy of
the tissue of the testes and subsequent infertility.)

We'll also remind you here about torsion of the testis.
This is not an injury, but is an acute and not too
uncommon condition of the testis that, if not treated
rapidly, can lead to the testis needing to be removed surgically. It typically occurs in boys in their teenage years and
young men, and is marked by the sudden onset of agonizing pain in the groin and lower abdomen, with
accompanying vomiting. The testis twists around on its
attachment to the spermatic cord like a yo-yo on a string,
thereby cutting off its own blood supply—if surgery is
not quickly performed, the testis dies and no longer
produces sperm or testosterone. Once this occurs on one
side, the other side is also prone to torsion so it is usual
for the surgeon to operate to fix the other testis firmly in
place as well.

Although not directly injuries to the penis or testes, we
must give some attention to spinal cord injuries because
they can very seriously impact on sexual functioning.

Jamal had everything going for him—a great job,
happy marriage, and a new home. He was in charge
of distribution for a large chain of stores and one day
was down in the truck bay checking out some details.
Before he could look up from his clipboard, he was
pinned against a wall by a fork lift truck. It was a
terrible accident that left Jamal paralyzed from the
waist down. Months of therapy ensued, with him
finally getting back enough control to walk with
special braces. He learned to control his bladder and

bowel functions. But damn, his new wife Elham had been so wonderful about all this and she was just so beautiful—he would get tremendously horny, but only in his mind. Nothing happened down below. Those connections from the brain to old Peter just didn't work anymore. Also, he and Elham really wanted children.

They talked it all over with Jamal's rehab specialist and it was decided that Jamal could use Viagra to produce an erection because he was young and in excellent health apart from the disabilities from the injury. With Elham physically stimulating him, this worked quite well. Jamal's nerves from his penis to and from the spinal cord were intact and functioning—it was the nerves higher up in the spinal cord which were permanently interrupted. The specialist also suggested trying a vacuum pump (we mentioned this device in Chapter 15). Jamal and Elham chose to use sometimes one and sometimes the other, and they were also provided with a vibrator device to produce ejaculation. Initially the specialist wasn't sure whether they could manage ejaculation during intercourse, so that Elham could conceive a child this way, but Elham soon learned to become very active in initiating their sexual episodes. The couple had already found alternative methods of expressing their love sexually and this was a welcome addition. Over and over, Jamal has said that he could not have recovered as he did—especially emotionally— without the fabulous support of Elham. Things have obviously gone well, because they are now expecting their first child.

DICK

Well, we warned you that this chapter was not for
the squeamish, but fortunately these injuries are not
common—in fact, have you ever heard of any except the
zipper pull among your friends?

CANCERS: "THE BIG C" 20

CANCER OF THE PENIS

Phil was in his seventies, ten years retired from the bank and very proud of his dahlias and his grandchildren. For some time he'd had an itch when he first emptied his bladder in the mornings, and then one day he noticed a small ulcer right on the tip of his old boy. A biopsy two days later showed that this was an early cancer of the skin of his glans, and the following week Phil underwent a partial penectomy, parting company with a good chunk of his old mate so that the tumor was completely excised.

Phil's wife died several years ago, so he just laughed when his urologist told him his sex life might be "compromised" and was more interested in knowing whether he'd still be able to pee standing up. This the urologist was able to achieve by fashioning a new urethral opening for Phil at the end of his new penis, which was shorter and stumpier than it had been, certainly, but was still recognizably a penis.

Andrew, a former patient of Michele's, was an engineer with a non-government agency in Africa in the early 1990s. He had always been a very handsome man with a very active sex life, and Africa was a good playground for him. One early morning, the previous night's sex partner fondled his penis and asked: "What's this?" "This" was a raised, firm little bump near the base of his penis that Andrew hadn't noticed because it was painless. He went that same morning to a doctor at the university hospital with which his group was associated. The lump was biopsied and the report was not good: Andrew had cancer of the penis. And the treatment involved amputation of the penis . . . without any time to get used to the idea.

Andrew flew to Switzerland for treatment and had both surgery and radiation therapy. While recuperating in a beautiful room overlooking a lake and mountains, Andrew made a startling decision: if he had to be without a penis, he would have a sex change and become a woman. (Needless to say, very few men choose this option, but this is a true story.) He did a lot of research and eventually flew to South Africa, where the necessary plastic surgery was done; this was after months of preparation with a psychologist and of taking female hormones, which he would now need to do for the rest of his life. Just before the surgery, Andrew legally changed his name to Andrea and told his family and those close friends who were not already aware.

Today, Andrew/Andrea is cancer-free and retired to a quiet life in a small Swedish town. Some of her new friends know her story, but no one questions this tall, handsome woman. Sex ... we don't know. Andrea isn't telling.

Sex-change operations are not common, but neither is cancer of the penis. Cancer of the penis is psychologically devastating, and unfortunately many men delay seeking health care early because of fear and a welter of conflicting emotions. No, they don't yet know what it is, but they do know something's going on with old Roger and it can't be good. The frequency of penile cancer varies throughout the world, accounting for only 0.4–0.6 percent of all malignancies in Europe and the United States, but 20–30 percent of all cancers diagnosed in men in Asia, Africa, and South America. The cancer rarely occurs in circumcised men and is thought to be associated with viruses, especially the papilloma or wart virus, taking up residence within the foreskin. This is still not completely proven, though there is much to support it and there are clearly also other, as yet unknown, factors involved. Because of the rarity of this cancer in men circumcised as infants, it is assumed that good hygienic practices (such as cleansing routinely and frequently under the foreskin in uncircumcised men) may also help prevent this. It is also known that there is an increase in cervical cancer in those women whose partners have had cancer of the penis, and human papilloma virus types 16 and 18 have been found in one-third of men who have penile cancer. While this has not been proven to be causative, it is certainly a strong association. The latest good news, however, is the possibility of a vaccine that will protect against these virus types.

Treatment of early small cancers may be possible with radiotherapy alone. More extensive cancers require surgery—yes, either partial or total amputation of your very best friend. In Andrew's case, because of the location of the tumor, his amputation had to be complete whereas for Phil, partial penectomy was sufficient. Surgery is usually followed by radiation of the lymph nodes in the surrounding areas, if they cannot be adequately removed during the surgery. It is imperative to seek treatment early—this means checking up on any unusual bumps or rashes or irritations on your penis—because untreated cancer of the penis spreads quickly and can lead to death within two years. It does not go away by itself. Nothing will replace a visit to your doctor as soon as you notice anything amiss.

Even when amputation needs to be complete or nearly so, later plastic surgery using skin grafts and prostheses can be used to reconstruct Dick. No, it won't be like it was—but with intensive rehabilitation and counseling, and possibly using one of the pump devices we mentioned in Chapter 15, erection and sometimes orgasm can still occur.

TESTICULAR CANCER

Nathan and Suzanne are both highly motivated people; they met in first year medical school and married after graduation. Now Nathan has just finished training as a pediatrician and Suzanne is doing a graduate course in public health. They are in their early thirties and, finally foreseeing an end to their formal education years, thought it was a good time to start a family. They decided that their anniversary was to be conception day and planned a romantic dinner at their favorite restaurant, followed by an early return to fresh sheets and soft music.

All went as planned until Suzanne was stroking Nathan's balls and her fingers lingered over an irregularity. Instantly, the instincts ingrained through years of training snapped into place and she began gently feeling his testis—the left one. Yes, there definitely was a lump there.

All thoughts of lovemaking flew out the window as Nathan and Suzanne discussed the possible implications of this lump. First thing the next morning, they went to the hospital and grabbed a urologist colleague (Dr. Cohen) to examine Nathan. Nathan had had surgery as a little fellow, to bring down a "floating testis." Dr. Cohen ordered an immediate ultrasound of Nathan's testis. This confirmed that the problem truly was in the testis, so next Nathan had a battery of blood tests, a CT scan of the abdomen, and a chest X-ray. The blood tests would look for tumor markers and all these tests were done to help stage the tumor. It is always assumed that any testicular mass is cancer until proven otherwise.

What about the baby who was to have been conceived that fateful night? Nathan was encouraged to have sperm banked so that, no matter what happened, he and Suzanne could start a family.

Our story has a happy ending. Nathan did indeed have testicular cancer, but it was discovered very early. He had the testis removed on that side, and eventually had a prosthesis put in so there was still a "ball" there. He also needed radiotherapy, but recovered completely. He and Suzanne now have two lovely little daughters, conceived by insemination with his frozen sperm.

Dermot also had testicular cancer. He was twenty-five at the time, and until then life had seemed near-perfect. He'd just finished a stint in the army, had found a job he liked in the construction industry, worked out in the gym, enjoyed a few beers at night with his friends, and had found a very special friend. In fact, he and Hal were about to start living together and come out to both families. Life was good. Then came the morning when he was in the shower as usual, and felt a little soft swelling in his right ball. After a few days of putting it off, he went to see his usual doc, who dispatched him straight away to a specialist urologist. Like Nathan, Dermot had a good outcome after surgery and radiotherapy, but noted that his energy level was different from before, and he did not have the same muscle strength as previously so he had to come up with a career change. Now Dermot is training to be a draftsman. The best thing has been Hal—he moved in and took care of Dermot through it all and really kept Dermot going, and they are still together.

Testicular cancer is rare, but is the most common cancer in young men. As illustrated by Nathan and Dermot, testicular cancer most commonly presents with a painless lump on one of the testes. Sometimes it will be accompanied by some swelling or pain in the scrotum.

It is a disease of younger men—generally ages fifteen through thirty-five—although it can occur at any age.

Symptoms of testicular cancer include the following:

- a lump in either testicle—may be any size;
- any enlargement of a testicle;
- a change in how the testicle feels (is it hard or bumpy?);
- a shrinking of the testis;
- pain or discomfort in the scrotum;
- fluid in the scrotum;
- a heavy feeling or dull ache in the groin or lower abdomen.

If you note any of the above, you should not delay in seeing your doctor. The good news is that testicular cancer, when diagnosed and treated promptly, has an excellent prognosis, with cure rates in excess of 95 percent. To be sure of these excellent results, of course, you need to be faithful with your follow-up appointments. The deaths that occur from testicular cancer these days tend to happen most often in those who do not keep going back to hear that they are OK. Young men tend to feel invulnerable and want to put distance between themselves and this brush with mortality. It is even better news that sterility is not always an outcome of treatment, although this is an individual matter. Fortunately, sexual function is usually preserved.

OTHER CANCERS
While it is not within our scope to discuss all of these in detail, we need to touch upon a few other cancers that can affect sexual functioning of your one-eyed snake.

Cancer of the prostate is the second most common non-skin cancer in men. There are many books and Web sites devoted to this topic, and you can seek them out for more in-depth information—see Appendix 3. Surgical removal of the prostate may be recommended for early cancer, especially in younger men, and is done as an open surgery through the area just north of the pubic bone. (The approach to the prostate gland through the urethra—the "trans-urethral resection," abbreviated as TUR or TURP, depending on where you live—may be used for diagnosis or to relieve obstruction if the bladder is blocked by the cancer.) The surgeon is always particularly careful not to damage the nerve plexus around the prostate but, even with all the good will in the world, this does happen—especially when the cancer is extensive and a wide excision needs to be done. If this happens, problems with getting Dick up may result. The best figures we've found show 30–40 percent of men are affected by erectile dysfunction after open prostatectomy. This is not likely to be improved by Viagra, but prostheses (penile implants) or pumps may be useful.

Also, as we mentioned previously, a sequel of prostate surgery through the urethra may be that the bladder no longer closes off during ejaculation, so the ejaculate does not spurt out through the urethra but instead passes into the bladder—"retrograde ejaculation." The sensation may therefore be a bit different than before surgery, but sex is still possible.

Some men will have erectile difficulties after prostate surgery not because of any physical damage, but because they are psychologically traumatized by the whole event.

This is quite common as well as completely under-standable—and responds well to a loving partner and some counseling.

Some of the same problems may arise from a TUR done for benign reasons—for example, a prostate big enough that you have to get up to pee six times per night and doing it takes forever. With this surgery there is no damage to the nerves, as in the open operation, but retrograde ejaculation and psychological consequences are common. Discuss all possibilities in depth with your doctor before any surgery to understand what your own particular risks are, and remember that hey! you are still alive, and healthy.

Cancer of the colon is common with both men and women and, if detected early, is eminently treatable. Early detec-tion is the key here and we urge each of you to utilize the screening methods available, especially where there is a family history of bowel cancer.

Remember that the nerves to the penis leave the spinal cord to come out of the lower vertebrae (see Figure 3.2) and they occupy the space on each side of the rectum as they pass forward to the penis. In surgery—especially extensive surgery of the lower bowel—these can be injured, resulting in an inability to raise the flag. This is much less likely to happen with an early cancer, confined to the inner bowel, so that's another good reason to do all the suggested screenings regularly. There are also various devices available that can be used during bowel surgery to locate and test the activity of the nerves that bring about erection, thus avoiding damage to them. More detail is beyond the scope of this book, but we urge you, if you are facing such surgery, not to hesitate to discuss the subject with your surgeon, if sexual functioning after your op is important to you—and why wouldn't it be? Your partner may also have an interest in knowing what to expect in this regard following your surgery.

Men who end up with colostomies following bowel surgery—usually for cancer, but sometimes for benign reasons—often have problems with body image and depression. This can adversely affect their sexuality, even when nerve function has not been damaged. Again, the role of the partner is critically important: a loving and sympathetic partner can make all the difference in the world. Counseling is also very helpful, and the various ostomy associations are very good for this.

Polyps and cancers of the bladder

These conditions, not rare, are beyond the scope of our book. But their presenting symptoms and signs—blood in the urine (hematuria) or blood coming from the urethra before or after peeing, and pain low down in the belly or burning while urinating—certainly involve Dick. So we'll emphasize here that any of the above symptoms should prompt a visit to your doctor to have it all checked out.

Bladder cancer may sometimes necessitate extensive surgery, with removal of the bladder required. This results in the wearing of a bag to collect the urine. Such surgery may damage the nerve supply to the penis and the wearing of the bag may damage self-esteem and body image. Either of these puts a serious damper on sexuality.

Radiotherapy for these various cancers, when indicated, may have a variable effect on sexual functioning. It is best to discuss your particulars with your doctor.

Obviously, finding out that you have cancer of any type or description is terrifying news and most, although not all, men are so happy to find they are alive and have a reasonable prognosis for the future that they are more than willing to explore other means of expressing their sexuality if necessary. Life takes on a whole new perspective.

21 CASTRATION: HISTORICAL CUSTOM CLIPS

Eunuchs bring to mind images from exotic tales: large beardless men, dressed in flowing harem trousers, sashed with brilliant cummerbunds, arms folded, guarding the entrance to the seraglio. Or leading a bevy of beauties, swathed in diaphanous and shimmering lengths of cloth, faces hidden from view, from their private quarters to the court of their master. Such is the stuff of tales . . . and of history.

Eunuchs were castrated men, used in the ancient lands of the Middle East, Egypt, India, and China to guard the high and holy, safeguard harems, and act as spies for their masters—"eunuch" is a Greek word meaning "guardian of the bed." There is mention of them in the Bible, and the panoply of ancient Egyptian gods included Seth, a eunuch. Many were castrated as children, specially selected for this purpose. The criteria varied with the culture. Others were slaves who had been captured and were for one reason or other thought to be good candidates; sometimes it was a method of subjugating an unruly enemy.

Just what is castration? It involves emasculating a man or boy, most commonly by cutting out his testes. Sometimes the whole penis was amputated as well (the "clean-shaven" eunuch), but this led to a higher-than-desired mortality rate, especially when it was done after puberty. Methods varied in various cultures, but it could be as simple as making a slit in the scrotum and cutting out the testes, or tying a cord very tightly around the base of the testes and allowing them to die from lack of blood supply. Sometimes the cord was of ceremonial color or material. Other practitioners simply crushed the testicles—*eeeeeowwhh!*

A distinction can be made between those castrated before puberty and those after. Prepubertal castration led to the distinctive habitus of a beardless man with a tendency to fat in the hips and belly, a higher voice, and a small penis, useless for anything but pissing. China's last imperial eunuch died in 1996 at the age of ninety-six; the average lifespan of eunuchs was longer than that of intact males. Those castrated after puberty, though, had fully developed penises and secondary sexual characteristics—body hair and muscle growth—and were generally capable of raising the flag and saluting a fair woman. Many married ladies of ancient Rome were said to favor the company of such eunuchs, since they were reliably sterile.

In the West, some early Christians castrated themselves in the name of celibacy as early as the third century. This was not condoned by the early Church, but by the 1500s, Pope Clement VII was greatly admiring of the high, pure voices of the *castrati* in the papal choir. The soaring high parts in liturgical music needed singers with appropriate voices and it was considered nigh on blasphemous for a woman to perform in church. Thus the *castrati*.

Young boys were selected (bought, stolen, seduced) to become *castrati*. They were then drugged with opium or spirits, immersed in a sensuously warm bath (remember, this was a time with no indoor plumbing!) and when their consciousness was dim enough, the testes were cut. This kept their voices high, although it did not guarantee that the boy would have a melodic singing voice.

With the advent of opera, *castrati* with good singing voices became the stuff of legends. They were the rock stars of their day, and all the hype and sexual frenzy that surrounds rock stars also attended them. Like the earlier post-pubertal eunuchs, many of them retained their sex drive and the ability to have an erection. Because of this, some became famous lovers, among them Farinelli.

Handel wrote music for the voice of Gaetano Guadagni, as did Gluck. Mozart's "Exultate, jubilate" was written for Venanzio Rauzzini. Meyerbeer was the last composer to write parts specifically for the male soprano and he wrote for Giovanni Velluti, who was famed for his coloratura and his outrageous manner of dress.

Castrati were replaced in theater by women, but survived longer in the Catholic Church. Alessandro Moreschi was the last of the famous *castrati* and was the only one ever to record. He died in 1922. The practice of castration in Western Europe was banned by Napoleon in 1802 and in the Catholic Church by Pope Leo XIII in 1878.

The next chapter in the saga of human castration began in 1869, with the publication of *Hereditary Genius* by Sir Francis Galton. Galton was much impressed by Darwin's theory of evolution and, in this pseudo-scientific paper, Galton concludes that nature produces the superior man, and that future changes in the human race could be engineered through careful breeding practices, much as is done in animal husbandry. Galton went on to coin the term "eugenics" as a science devoted to the improvement of the human stock by enabling the superior races and strains of blood to prevail over the unsuitable. Unsuitable included mentally ill, poor, criminals, and people of color. Galton's views stirred a brisk intellectual debate.

In the United States, Galton's hypotheses were embraced enthusiastically by many titans of industry and the intelligentsia of the ivory towers. Harvard-educated and Carnegie-funded Dr. Charles Davenport led the call to not just sterilize, but castrate, the mentally ill and all other misfits. This was taken to heart and a spate of academic articles appeared in the prestigious medical journals, all supporting the application of eugenics, a brave new science.

By 1907, Indiana passed the first compulsory sterilization law; soon thirty U.S. states had such laws. The laws basically called for the sterilization of all people felt to be "social misfits." Indiana may have been the first, but California led the way in actually implementing these laws and the U.S. Supreme Court found that compulsory sterilization was indeed constitutional. By 1945, more than 45,000 Americans had been sterilized under these laws. Indeed, Hitler's eugenists looked to the American model. They, however, carried things further—as history attests.

After World War II, compulsory sterilization or castration for social misfits was largely dropped. The exception to this was, and is, the application to sex offenders. This is controversial and subject to fierce debate, but still favored by some of the perpetrators as well as some lawmakers, criminologists, and scientists. Castration is now chemical, using drugs that block the pituitary hormones that stimulate the testes' production of testosterone. An article in the *New England Journal of Medicine* in 1998 indicated that the use of chemical castration provided therapeutic value and substantially reduced the recidivism of sex offenders, especially pedophiles. As we write, five American states have laws providing for mandatory chemical castration for pedophiles.

There are times when castration is done for strictly medical reasons. As already discussed, castration is a definitive treatment for cancer of the penis, in the sense that some or part of the penis (though not the testes) needs to be amputated to remove the tumor. However, penile cancer is pretty rare. It is also usual to offer plastic surgery to reconstruct the penis after amputation for cancer-related reasons. Castration is also a necessary part of the treatment for testicular cancer, which is not common, but is the most common cancer in young men between the ages of fifteen and thirty-four. In this case, usually only one testis is removed and post-operation synthetic testosterone can be given if needed. Chemical or hormonal castration is part of the treatment regimen for prostatic cancer, because testosterone and other androgens stimulate the growth of the cancer, but it is not an inevitable part of the treatment.

As you can see, castration has historically been more of a cultural and societal phenomenon than it has been a medical one.

DICK NUTRITION GUIDE 22

There is much controversy today over what is the best diet, with the old food pyramid being thrown out the window and nothing in particular replacing it. These guidelines incorporate the various pieces of nutrition research about which there are no quibbles and also give you an easy and palatable way to eat for health.

1. DO eat 5 to 10 servings of fruits and vegetables each day. These taste good, fill the empty pit, and are full of various pigments, vitamins, minerals, and other goodies that ward off disease. No kidding—for example, it has been shown that eating about 5 servings per week of cooked tomato products can help prevent prostate cancer. With no downside.
2. DO eat 2 to 3 servings of around 3 ounces (about the size of your palm) of protein every day. This can be animal protein, like lean meats, fish, or fowl, dried beans (cooked, of course), dairy products such as cottage or farmer's cheese or hard cheeses, or soybean products, such as tofu. Dairy products are also essential for calcium, to keep your bones healthy.

3. DO eat grain products to tie things together. The old guidelines specified 6 to 11 servings, and this was a little high for people who tend to roundness or are more sedentary. The big proviso here is that we're talking about whole-grain products, not your favorite cake or white dinner roll. Rice and millet work, as does oatmeal and a good hefty whole-meal bread. Grains give you fiber and many vitamins and are an important part of a balanced diet, but too much of these good things will make you fat.

4. DO eat some fat. We need the essential fatty acids in fat to make our own anti-inflammatory substances and as precursors for many hormones. What is important is the type of fat. The fats found in fish, nuts, seeds, and olives are good for you. Again, too much of a good thing is no longer good, but current thinking is that up to about 20 percent good fat content in the diet is acceptable. Lean meats are also acceptable sources of fat. Go easy on the butter (perhaps combine $1/4$ pound of butter with $1/3$ cup of light oil and make your own spread) and avoid fried foods. Margarine is dicey because it contains fatty acids in a form called trans fatty acids and these are unhealthy.

5. A small, consistent amount of alcohol has been shown to be healthy for the heart. Note that the frequency of use matters more than amounts, so that you could use a tablespoon of wine each day and derive the benefits: you don't need to become a regular at the local bar.

6. Calcium supplements have been shown to have a protective effect on the bowel and are cheap and easy. Again, like the alcohol, it isn't dose-related, so a little will do.

7. The benefits of taking a multiple vitamin each day have also been demonstrated. Just remember to look for one that contains no iron—men do not need iron above and beyond what is in the diet.

When all is said and done, a healthy Dick is a happy one and your buddy is dependent upon the general health of the rest of you.

23 A DICK-TIONARY OF SLANG

In Nicaragua, a penis is lovingly referred to as "la paloma," or dove. A few years ago, the government was promoting appropriate transportation by importing a large number of bicycles from China. The brand name emblazoned across the cross-bars was "La Paloma Volente," or the flying . . . dove. Many chuckles and a few red faces ensued.

We're sure our list of slang terms and euphemisms for the penis is far from complete, but still it's a long list. In fact, we've found nearly 400 of these endearments. (This is in sharp contrast to words, slang and otherwise, for the vagina, of which only about a dozen exist amongst English speakers. Clearly the subject holds enormous interest for the guys.) As you'll have noticed, we've tried to use many of these throughout the book.

Mostly, we'll let these terms stand on their own, without trying to be too clever or cute, as many people use them in a very serious and straightforward manner. But we couldn't resist a few comments along the way. The same term can sometimes be used in several ways—there's a fine difference that we're sure you'll appreciate between "he has a big prick" and "he is a big prick," for example. Here we go . . .

Aaron's rod
Action man
Arrow (in fact, all weapons are
    popular)
Artillery
Assailant
Baby maker
Bag boy
Bag of tricks
Bald root
Ballcock
Balls (not strictly penis)
Banana
Banger (also Big banger)
Battering ram
Beak
Beef bayonet (also Hot beef)
Bell boy
Bellpull
Best man
Big banana
Big Bob
Big boy
Big honcho, big bamboo
Big man on campus
Big one
Blade
Blind Bob
Blind eye
Blind man
Bludgeon
Bob
Boner
Broom handle
Bush beater
Candle
Cannon
Captain Standish
Captain, cavalier
Carnal man

Carrot
Chap (also Old chap)
Cherry picker
Chilli (with various adjectives)
Chopper
Chucker, chuck
Clothes pin or peg
Club
Cock, cocksman
Codpiece
Crack hunter
Cranny hunter
Creamsickle
Creamstick
Crimson bird (a red paloma?)
Crown jewels
Cuckoo
Cucumber (or veggie of your
    choice)
Cupid's torch
Cyclops
Dick (of course!) and aka Moby
Dickety boy
Diddler
Didgeridoo
Dildo (also a fake penis)
Ding-a-ling
Dingbat
Ding-dong, dingle, dingle-dangle
Dingus
Diplomat
Dipstick
Disturber of the peace (piece)
Do-funny
Do-gooder
Donger, dong
Donut puncher
Doodle
Dork
Dragon

DICK

Dribbler
Drumstick
Dum-dum
Eel
Egghead
End piece
Engine
Equipment
Erogenous part
Extension
Faithful friend
Faithful servant
Family jewel
Fanny rat
Father confessor
Fellow, also fella, little fella and
    old fellow/fella
Fiddle bow
Finger
Fingamajig
Flip-flop
Flute
Flying blowtorch
Flying dick
Fornicator
Frankfurter
Freudian tip (not bad!)
Frigger
Fruit
Fucker (and more along these
    lines which we'll leave to your
    imagination)
Gap stopper
Gem
General
Generator
Gentle tickler
Giggle stick
Girl pleaser
Girlometer

Gold digger
Goober
Gooseneck
Grand masterpiece
Gravy giver
Greenstick
Grinding tool
Grunt iron
Hambone
Headlight
Hermit
Hoe handle
Hooded bandit
Horn
Hose
Hot pudding
Hot rod, hot dog
Implement
Instrument
Irish root
Iron
Jack
Jade scepter
Jade stem
Jerking iron
Jerktown
John Thomas
Johnson
Joint
Jokester
Jolly Roger
Joy knob
Joy stick
Juice man
Junior
Kit and caboodle
Knob
Knocker
Kojak, Yul Brynner
    (or any bald-headed man)

Ladies' delight
Lamp of life (really!)
Lead joint
Lead pipe clincher
Leg
Life preserver
Lingam
Lip splitter
Little man, little fireman
Lizard
Lollipop
Love gun, love trumpet, love tool, love sausage, etc., etc.
Love sword, love pole, love pistol
Lunchbox (the whole package, we guess)
Magic wand
Manhood mushroom
Marrowbone
Meat (also man meat)
Member (gold and other colors)
Milkman
Missile, heat-seeking missile
Monk, also monkey
Mousie
Mr. Floppy (who'd admit to that one?)
Mr. Happy
Mr. Jones Mulligan
Mr. Know-it-all
Muscle of love, also inflatable muscle of love
My affair
My business end
My little buddy
Nag
Nature's masterpiece
Nature's scythe
Nice little piece of possibility
Nine-inch knocker (above the national average, see "size")
Noodle
Nose
Nuthouse
Old blind Bob
Old boy, old sausage, and many similar endearments
Old Horny
Old Jack
Old Slimy
One-eyed Jack
One-eyed trouser snake
Organ of generation
Oscar
Peacemaker
Pecker
Pee pee
Peewee
Pego
Pendulum
Percolator
Percy (for pointing at the porcelain)
Perker up
Peter, Pete, old Pete
Phallus
Pikestaff
Pile driver
Pilgrim's staff
Pillar, pillar of ivory
Pioneer
Pipe
Pipe organ
Pisser
Pistol
Piston
Plank
Plaything
Pleasure machine
Plough

DICK

Plug
Plum picker
Point
Poker
Pole
Poontagger
Pork sword
Potent regiment
Potz, putz
Priapus
Prick
Pride and joy
Privates
Proboscis
Prong
Pud (as in "pulling the pud")
Pump
Purple-headed love warrior
Purple people eater (a generational
    thing)
Quartermaster
Quim
Rabbit
Radish (veggies *again*)
Rainstick
Ramrod, rod
Randy mole
Reamer
Rector
Red cap
Red-hot poker
Reverend
Richard (Dick to his friends!)
Roger and out
Roger (also Roger Ramjet)
Rolling pin
Rooster
Ruffian
Rump splitter
Saint Peter

Salami, old salami
Sausage (fries with that?)
Sceptre
Schlong
Schmuck
Screwdriver
Seat of strength
Semi-automatic
Sexing piece
Shaft
Short arm
Slug
Snake in the grass
Solicitor general
Spear of love
Spindle
Spunker
Stalk
Stallion
Steed
Stem
Stick
Sting
Stud poker
Stump
Stumper
Submarine
Sword
Tailpipe
The professor
The Right Honorable Member
    for Underpants (really?)
Thing
Third leg
Thorn in the flesh
Thumb of love
Thunderstick
Tickler
Todger
Tonsil tickler

Tool
Torch
Trickster
Trigger
Trouser snake, trouser serpent, trouser wasp
Truncheon
Tube of lipstick
Unicorn
Utensil
Veined sausage
Wanger, wing wang
Wanker
Water spout
Water works
Wazoo

Weapon
Wedding tackle
Wee wee, weenie, weiner, woo woo
Whip
Whore pipe
Wife's best friend
Wig-wag, wick, winkle
Willie
Winkie, wee willie winkie, winky
Worm
Yang
Yard (you wish!)
Yard stick (ditto)
Yum-Yum
Zeppelin

And for the testicles: balls, nuts, hairy eggs, goolies, googlies, beanbags, happy sack, 'nads (short for gonads), jelly beans, and Easter eggs.

These are but a few of the many terms affectionately used for your favorite male attributes. Each language has its own long list.

Some lists of information follow, which we hope may be helpful to you. We hope also that, regardless of whether you think of Dick as a scepter, a sausage, or a purple-headed love warrior, you have found our book helpful, and fun. Certainly, writing it for you has given us quite a rise.

APPENDIX 1: INFECTIONS AND SEXUALLY TRANSMITTED DISEASES

Disease	Cause	Incubation	Organs affected	Symptoms	Complications	Diagnosis	Treatment	Prevention
Gonorrhea	Neisseria gonorrhea, a bacterium	3–10 days	Urethra, cervix, uterus tubes, others	Pain on peeing, discharge	PID, sterility, arthritis	Swab for DNA, probe, culture	Antibiotics	Condoms, abstinence
Herpes	Herpes simplex, type 2	2–20 days sometimes longer	Vagina, vulva, penis, mouth, anus, throat	Flu-like, tingling, shallow, painful ulcers	Rare	Swab and/or blood tests for antibody	Supportive, acyclovir, valacyclovir	Condoms, abstinence, C-section for baby, vaccine in research
Genital warts	Human Papilloma Virus (HPV)	Variable	Penis scrotum, perineum, vulva, cervix, anus	Warty growths, itch	Cancer of penis or cervix—types 16, 18, 31	Viral testing Pap smears	imiquimod, podophyllo-toxin, surgery	condoms, abstinence, vaccines in research
Syphilis	Treponema pallidum	2–6 weeks	Penis, cervix, vulva, skin, mucous membranes, heart, blood vessels, brain	Painless hard ulcer, rash, malaise, psychiatric symptoms	Death from neurological, cardiovascular effects	Blood test, biopsy	Antibiotics: important to take entire course	Condoms, abstinence

Disease	Cause	Incubation	Organs affected	Symptoms	Complications	Diagnosis	Treatment	Prevention
Chlamydia	chlamydia trachomatis a bacterium	variable	urethra, anus, vagina, cervix, tubes, uterus, ovaries	often none can be burning discharge	infertility PTD	DNA probes from urethra, anus, vagina, cervix	antibiotics	condoms abstinence
hepatitis B	hepatitis B virus	4 weeks to 6 months	Liver, brain	Malaise, vomiting, jaundice	Chronic hepatitis, cancer risk, death	Blood tests	Supportive, liver transplantation	hepatitis B vaccine, condoms, hygiene
Trichomonas	Trichomonad parasites	1–4 weeks	Urethra, vagina, bladder	Painful peeing, burning, discharge	None	Wet slide prep	Flagyl	Condoms
Granuloma inguinale	Donovania granulomatis bacterium	8–12 weeks	All genital area, lower abdomen, buttocks	Painful, oozing ulcer	Secondary infection by another bacteria	Scrapings or biopsy	Antibiotics	Condoms
Chancroid	Hemophilus ducreyii bacterium	3–5 days	Penis, vulva, cervix, perineum	Painful, oozing ulcer, swollen and tender lymph nodes	Scarring, secondary infection	Culture from ulcers	Antibiotics, drainage of lymph nodes	Condoms, abstinence

Disease	Cause	Incubation	Organs affected	Symptoms	Complications	Diagnosis	Treatment	Prevention
TB	Myco-bacterium tuberculosis	Variable	Testes, epididymis, many others	Firm mass that may break through skin	Generalized TB	Biopsy	Anti-TB drugs	Good general health
Mumps	Mumps virus	18 days	Testes, parotid gland	Swelling pain, fever	Atrophy of testes, infertility	Physical examination, blood	Supportive	Mumps vaccine
Filariasis	Wucheria bancrofti parasite	4–12 months	Lymphatics, lung	Scrotal pain and swelling, fever	Irreversible swelling of genitals, elephantiasis	Blood and skin tests, ultrasound	Anti-parasite drugs	Mosquito control
HIV	Human immuno-deficiency virus	Variable	Immune system	Malaise, fatigue, infections, headaches cancers, etc.	Death	Blood test	No cure, drug "cocktails" manage disease	Safe sex
Urinary tract infection	Bacteria from bowel, skin	Variable	Bladder, kidneys, urethra	Pain in abdomen, burning on peeing	Kidney infection and damage	Urine specimen for lab culture	Antibiotics	Treat obstructions to flow of urine

APPENDIX 2: FAMILY PLANNING/PLANNED PARENTHOOD CLINICS AND SEXUAL HEALTH CLINICS

UNITED STATES

International Planned Parenthood
    Federation
120 Wall Street, 9th Floor
New York, NY 10005
Ph: 212 248 6400
Fax: 212 248 4221
Email: info@ippfwhr.org
Web: www.ippfwhr.org

Planned Parenthood
Phone for nearest clinic:
    1 800 230 PLAN

American Foundation for
    Urologic Disease
1128 North Charles Street
Baltimore, MD 21201
Ph: 410 468-1800
Fax: 410 468-1808
Toll free: 800 242-2383
Web: www.afud.org

Men's Health Network
PO Box 75972
Washington, D.C. 20013
Ph: 202 543-6461
Web:
    www.menshealthnetwork.org
Men's health
www.menshealth.about.com

Men's Journal
1290 Avenue of the Americas
New York, NY 10104-0298
Web: www.mensjournal.com

Men's health issues posted by the
    University of Texas-Houston
    Medical School
Web: www.medic.med.uth.tmc.
    edu/ptnt/00000391.htm

FDA site on birth control
Web: www.fda.gov/opacom/
    lowlit/brthcon.html

AFRICA

Africa Region International
  Planned Parenthood
Madison Insurance House
Upper Hill Road/Ngong Road
Nairobi, Kenya
Ph: 254 (2) 720 280
Fax: 254 (2) 726 596
Email: info@ippfaro.org

ARAB WORLD

Arab World Regional Office
  International Planned
  Parenthood
2 Place Virgile
Notre Dame
Tunis, Tunisia 1082
Ph: 216 216 71 847 344
Fax: 216 216 71 788 661
Email: awro@ippf.intl.tn

ASIA

South Asia Regional Office
  International Planned
  Parenthood Federation

IPPF, Regent's College
Inner Circle, Regent's Park
London, NW1 4NS
Ph: 44 (20) 7487 7977
Fax: 44 (20) 7487 7970
Email: sarinfo@ippf.org

AUSTRALIA

Australian Men's Health
  Network
  Web:
  www.members.ozemail.com.au

Dubbo FPA Health Centre
221 Darling St,
Dubbo, NSW 2830
Ph: 02 6885 1544

Fairfield FPA Health
  Multicultural Services
356 the Horsley Drive,
Fairfield, NSW 2165
Ph: 02 9754 1322

FPA Chatswood
47 Hercules St,
Chatswood, NSW 2067
Ph: 02 9415 2700

FPA Health
328–336 Liverpool Rd,
Ashfield, NSW 2131
Ph: 02 9716 6099
Fax: 02 9716 6164
Web: www.fpahealth.org.au

FPA Healthline:
  1 300 658 886

Hurstville FPA Health Centre
12 The Avenue,
Hurstville, NSW
Ph: 02 9579 7722

Men's health
Web: www.mannet.com.au
Web: www.noah-health.org

Newcastle FPA
15–19 Queen St,
Cooks Hill, NSW
Ph: 02 4929 4485

DICK

Sexual Health and Family
   Planning Australia
Suite 4 Construction House
217 Northbourne Avenue,
Turner, ACT 2601
Ph: 02 6230 5255
Fax: 02 6230 5344
Web: www. fpa.net.au

Warehouse Youth Health Centre
13 Reserve St,
Penrith, NSW 2750
Ph: 02 4721 8330

Wollongong FPA Health Centre
1A Dension St,
Wollongong, NSW 2500
Ph: 02 4226 5816
Web: www.actonline.com.au/fpa

CANADA
European Network, International
   Planned Parenthood
146 rue Royale
Brussels, 1000
Ph: 32 (2) 250 09 50
Fax: 32 (2) 250 09 69
Email: info@ippfen.org
Web: www.ippfen.org

Planned Parenthood Federation of
   Canada
1–430 Nicholas
Ottawa, Ontario K1N 7B7
Ph: 613 241 4474
Fax: 613 241 7550
Email: admin@ppfc.ca
Web: www.ppfc.ca

IRELAND
EveryWoman Centre
5/7 Cathal Brugha Street
Dublin 1
Ph: 01 872 7088
Fax: 01 836 4533

IFPA National Office
Solomon's House
42A Pearse St
Dublin 2
Ph: 01 474 0944
Fax: 01 474 0945
Email: post@ifpa.ie
Web: www.ifpa.ie

NEW ZEALAND
New Zealand Family Planning
   Association (FPANZ)
Queen Street Centre
Level 4 Garico Commercial
   Building
109 Queen St
Central City, Auckland, NZ
Ph/Fax: 09 379 0657
Free number: 0800 372 5463
Web: www.fpanz.org.nz

UNITED KINGDOM
Contraceptive Education Service
   Hotline
Ph: 0845 310 1334

Engender Health
   Web:
   www.engenderhealth.org/ia/
   wwm/index.html

Family Health International
Web: www.fhi.org

FPA
Web: www.fpa.org

Marie Stopes Centres
Ph: 44 (I) 207 574 7400
Fax: 44 (I) 207 574 7417

National AIDS Helpline
Ph: 0800 567123

NHS Direct
Ph: 0845 4647

LISTINGS OF CERTIFIED SEXUAL THERAPISTS
Web: www.sextherapist.org.uk
Web: www.SEXHELP.org

APPENDIX 3:
REFERENCES,
RESOURCES, AND
FURTHER READING

ARTICLES

Legge, Kate and Minichiello, V. "Sex and Drugs and Rocking Chairs," University of New England School of Health Sciences, quoted in *The Australian Weekend Magazine*, 31 Aug 2002

Morley, J. E., Patrick, P. and Perry H.M.P. III, "Could it be Low Testosterone?," Dept of Geriatric Medicine, St. Louis University. Website: www.slu.edu/adam/maletquiz.pdf

Tiemstra, J. D. "Factors affecting the circumcision decision," *Journal of the American Board of Family Practice*, Jan–Feb 1999, 12:16–20

BOOKS

Barrett, David M. M.D. (ed.) (2000) *Mayo Clinic on Prostate Health: Answers from the World-Renowned Mayo Clinic on Prostate Inflammation, Enlargement, Cancer*, Kensington Publishing Corp.

Chang, Jolan (1993) *The Tao of Love and Sex*, New York, NY: Viking Press.

Chia, Mantak et al (1997) *The Multi-Orgasmic Man: Sexual Secrets Every Man Should Know*, Harper San Francisco, San Francisco, CA

Danielou, Alain (1995) *The Complete Kama Sutra: The First Unabridged Modern Translation of the Classic Indian Text*, Rochester, VT: Inner Traditions International, Ltd.

——— (1995) *The Phallus: Sacred Symbol of Male Creative Power*, Inner Traditions Int'l, Rochester, VT

Friedman, David M. (2001) *A Mind of Its Own: A Cultural History of the Penis*, Free Press, New York, NY

Friend, D. and Morely, S. (2000) *Puppetry of the Penis: The Ancient Australian Art of Genital Origami*, Corgi/Transworld Publishing, London, UK

Gore, Margaret (1997) *The Penis Book*, Allen & Unwin, Sydney, Australia

Hamilton, T. (2002) *Skin Flutes and Velvet Gloves: A Collection of Facts and Fancies, Legends and Oddities about the Body's Private Parts*, St. Martin's Press, New York, NY

Johnston, Jack (2001) *Male Multiple Orgasm: Step-by-Step* (4th Ed). Audio CD.

Jones, Derek Llewelyn (1999) *Every Man*, Oxford University Press, Oxford

Junot, Dan (1999) *Stop Premature Ejaculation and Learn to Control Male Orgasm*, Center for Special Services

Kinsey, Alfred C. (1948) *Sexual Behaviour in the Human Male*, Saunders, Philadelphia

Madaras, Lynda et al (2000) *What's Happening to My Body? Book for Boys: A Growing Up Guide for Parents and Sons*, New Market Press, New York, NY

Marks, Sheldon M.D. and Moul, Judd (1999) *Prostate and Cancer: A Family Guide to Diagnosis, Treatment and Survival*, Perseus Publishing, Cambridge, MA

Masters, William and Johnson, Virginia (1966) *Human Sexual Response*, Lippincott, Williams & Wilkins Publisher, Philadelphia

Natural Penis Enlargement: New methods of avoiding and curing impotence, premature ejaculation, and erectile dysfunction safely and inexpensively. NEW secrets that your doctor won't tell you, No Pumps, No Pills and No Gadgets (2002), Platinum Millennium Publishing

Newman, Alfred J. (1999) *Beyond Viagra: Plain Talk about Treating Male and Female Sexual Dysfunction*, Starrhill Press, Washington, DC

Norton, Bret (ed.) (2002) *Shunga: The Essence of Japanese Pillow-Book Eroticism.* Astrology Publishing House.

Parsons, A. and Black, J. (1990) *Facts and Phalluses: A Collection of Bizarre and Intriguing Truths, Legends and Measurements*, St. Martin's Press, New York, NY

Simon, H. B. and Greenfield, H. [illustrator] (2002) *The Harvard Medical School Guide to Men's Health*, Free Press, New York, NY

DICK

Steidle, Christopher P. and Mulcahy, John J. (1999) *The Impotence Sourcebook*, McGraw Hill/Contemporary Books, New York, NY

Strum, S. B. and Pogliano, D. (2000) *A Primer on Prostate Cancer: The Empowered Patient's Guide*, Life Extension Media, Southbury, CT

Walsh, Patrick M.D. and Farrar Worthington, Janet (2002) *Dr. Patrick Walsh's Guide to Surviving Prostate Cancer*, Warner Books, New York, NY

Watters, G. and Carroll, S. (2002) *Your Penis: A User's Guide*, Urology Publications, Port Macquarie, NSW, Australia

Winks, Cathy and Semans, Anne (2002) *The Good Vibrations Guide to Sex: The Most Complete Sex Manual Ever Written*, San Francisco, CA: Cleis Press.

INDEX